W9-BZO-617

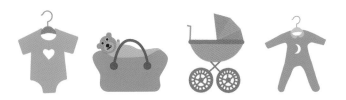

the Baby book

LONDON, NEW YORK, MUNICH, MELBOURNE, AND DELHI

Senior Editor Nikki Sims
Senior Art Editor Jane Ewart
Project Editors Becky Alexander, Claire Cross,
Joanna Edwards
Project Art Editors Stephen Bere, Hannah Moore,
Claire Patané
Jacket Design Assistant Rosie Levine
Production Editor Sarah Isle
Production Controller Seyhan Esen
Creative Technical Support Sonia Charbonnier
New Photography Ruth Jenkinson
Managing Editor Penny Smith
Senior Managing Art Editor Marianne Markham
Publisher Mary Ling
Creative Director Jane Bull
US Senior Editor Shannon Beatty
US Editor Jane Perlmutter
US Consultant Lisa Fields

Our consultants: Judith Barac and Dawn Woolacott.
Our team of writers: Shaoni Bhattacharya, Claire Cross, Carol
Dyce, Kate Ling, Susannah Marriott, Karen Sullivan, and Jo Wiltshire.

First American Edition, 2013

Published in the United States by

DK Publishing

375 Hudson Street

New York, New York 10014

13 14 15 16 17   10 9 8 7 6 5 4 3 2 1

001—184553—February/2013

Copyright © 2013 Dorling Kindersley Limited

All rights reserved

Without limiting the rights under copyright reserved above, no part of
this publication may be reproduced, stored in or introduced into a
retrieval system, or transmitted, in any form, or by any means (electronic,
mechanical, photocopying, recording, or otherwise), without the prior
written permission of both the copyright owner and the above publisher
of this book.

Published in Great Britain by Dorling Kindersley Limited.

A catalog record for this book is available from the Library of
Congress.

ISBN 978-1-4654-0192-2

DK books are available at special discounts when purchased in bulk for
sales promotions, premiums, fund-raising, or educational use. For details,
contact: DK Publishing Special Markets, 375 Hudson Street, New York,
New York 10014 or SpecialSales@dk.com.

Printed and bound by in China by South China Printing Co. Ltd.

Discover more at **www.dk.com**

contents

With baby on
board, life will
never be the same
again—and that is
a very good thing.

The road to *parenthood*

Congratulations! You're pregnant, and what's more, you're going to be a parent! You are now on a path that will bring new experiences, abilities, thoughts, emotions, and especially love. It's going to be one interesting journey.

One advantage of pregnancy taking nine long months is that you and your partner get the chance to come to terms with how life is about to change forever. You can plan for the delivery, shop for the baby, talk about the future, and make the most of your kid-free time together. Now is the time to read up and get ready.

Whether you are newly pregnant, or on your second or third pregnancy, you'll find that there is plenty to think about, and routine doctor appointments, choosing a stroller, and arranging your maternity leave can sometimes eclipse the incredible reality that you are carrying a new life within you, and that your body is nuturing that life.

The Baby Book is all about enjoying pregnancy and parenthood, while also coming to grips with the essentials so that you can take this incredible life stage all in your stride. It's reassuring to know, for instance, that emotions can swing between elation and blind panic within a matter of moments—and that is entirely normal.

{ A sound knowledge of what the next nine months hold, paves the way for a positive and happy pregnancy. }

This book informs rather than alarms parents-to-be, and offers glimpses into how pregnancy and birth are embraced by cultures around the world. Most of all, it helps you to enjoy this exciting stage of life.

Baby on Board takes you on a chronological journey through pregnancy, celebrating the amazing way your body adapts and the astonishing developments of your baby. Dip into topics, such as Does age matter?, The risk roller coaster, What do babies do all day?, and Will I get stretch marks?

Deep Breaths explores labor from a psychological and a physical perspective, so that you and your partner feel as ready as possible for the big day.

The Baby Book presents you with the facts and leaves you to make the decisions. Throughout, the book addresses the wider picture: that you are parents and what this means for you both. From cravings to being a birth partner, we give you facts and ideas to help you enjoy your pregnancy and look forward to the arrival of your baby.

Your baby
is the size of...

You're at the beginning of an incredible stage of life that will see your body undergo dramatic changes. From the moment of conception your baby grows at an extraordinary rate, from a tiny speck to a size comparable to a watermelon!

It all starts the size of a pinhead...

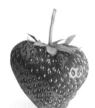
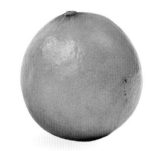
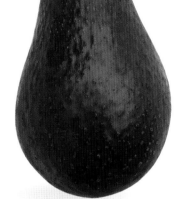

Weeks 1 to 6

From the first half hour of life, your baby is as small as a pinprick; by three weeks, the size of a grain of rice; and within six weeks, the size of a peanut. But amazing things are happening: her body, nose, and eyes are taking shape.

Week 8

By this time, your baby will look recognizably human, although partly transparent and about the size of a strawberry. Her tongue and some teeth are forming, and her heart has started beating.

Week 12

At the end of the first trimester, your baby has grown to the size of a lime or plum. By now her skeleton is almost complete, though it's made of cartilage not bone, and she can curl her toes and open and close her fingers.

Week 16

Now the size of an avocado, your baby has become quite active. She can make intricate movements such as clench her fists, suck her thumb, make facial expressions, and grasp the umbilical cord. She begins to hear sounds.

Week 8
Baby is
⅔in (1.6cm)

Week 12
Baby is 2in
(5cm)

Week 16
Baby is 4¾in
(12cm)

Week 18
Baby is 5½in
(14cm)

Week 20
Baby is 10in
(25cm)

0cm Average baby length from crown to rump.   **10cm**   **20cm** Average baby length from crown to heel.

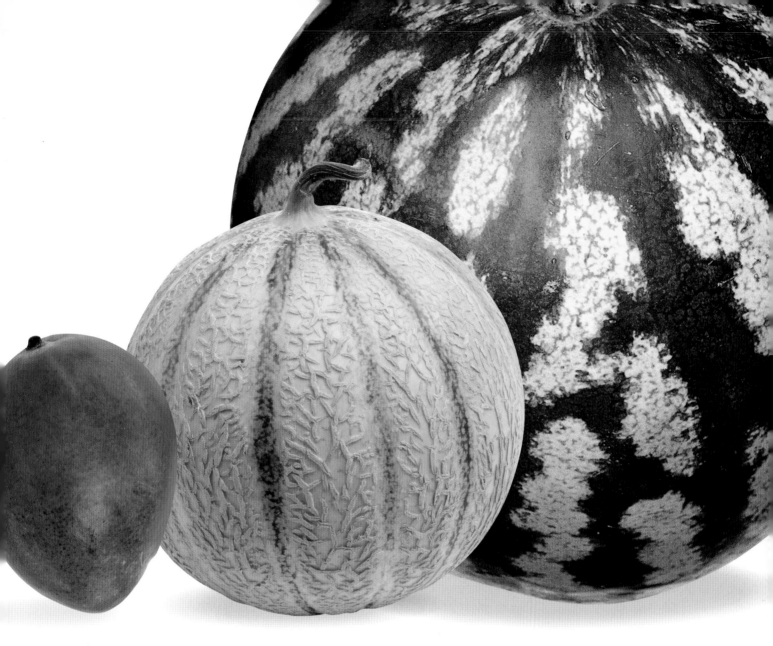

Week 20

You'll start to feel your baby's activity levels rise now that she's about the size of a large mango. Her legs have grown substantially and are now longer than her arms—she looks much more like the baby you'll meet.

Week 24

Your baby's eyes have opened, and she ingests large quantities of amniotic fluid, which are then excreted via the placenta. Her lungs practice breathing movements, but are still immature. She's about the size of a cantaloupe.

Week 30

Although your baby has less room to move around now, you'll feel sharper movements from her elbows and knees more. She is roughly the size of a medium-sized pumpkin and spends most of her time curled up sleeping and dreaming.

Weeks 38 to 40

During the final weeks of your pregnancy your baby will grow rapidly, ending up the size of a small watermelon. She can recognize your voice and her body is now preparing to deal with the outside world.

  Week 22
Baby is 11 in
(28 cm)

Week 26
Baby is 14 in
(36 cm)

 Week 30
Baby is 15¾ in
(40 cm)

 Week 34
Baby is 18 in
(46 cm)

Week 38
Baby is 20 in
(50 cm)

30 cm   40 cm   50 cm

And baby makes *three*

The arrival of your baby brings with it the extraordinary realization that from now on, with every word and action, you are shaping your child into a unique human being. It's quite a responsibility.

In the early days of parenthood you may find yourself wondering what on earth you have gotten yourself into. How do couples manage to look beyond the fatigue, feeding, financial cost, and responsibility, and still decide that parenthood was ever a good idea?

The resounding answer from parents is that the rewards are infinite and far outweigh the downside. From the pride you experience at having created this precious new life, to the excitement you feel when your child babbles his first word, having a child brings more fun to your life, as well as new depth and purpose. And now you are embarking on a whole new journey of discovery as you learn to become a parent—as well as retain some of the old you.

A Mini Miracle looks at life with a brand-new baby from the very first moments you hold him through to how best to burp him and give him his first bath. It looks at the experience of parenting around the world (there are many different right ways to do things), and addresses questions that come up on the way: How do I get my baby to sleep? Can I leave him alone? How do I know if I'm stimulating him enough? Or too much? And that's just the early stuff.

Hello, Gorgeous! and Thinking Big then explore how life changes when you have a walking and talking toddler and then child on your hands. Whether you need advice on behavioral issues, prompts on things to consider, such as a regular babysitter, or ideas of what to feed your child, these sections offer plenty of food for thought.

Part of being a parent is realizing that as time goes by, your child keeps changing, and no matter how many mini victories you celebrate —the diverted tantrums, the bedtime tears that fade— another new challenge will rise to take its place. Your child is learning to be a person just as you are learning to be a parent.

And just when you thought you were getting the hang of parenthood, it might be time to bring another baby into the mix. Expanding your Family looks at the importance (or not) of birth order, sibling relationships, and life with two or more children. Just to keep you on your toes.

> Every family does things differently. There is much we can learn from each other, but most is up to you!

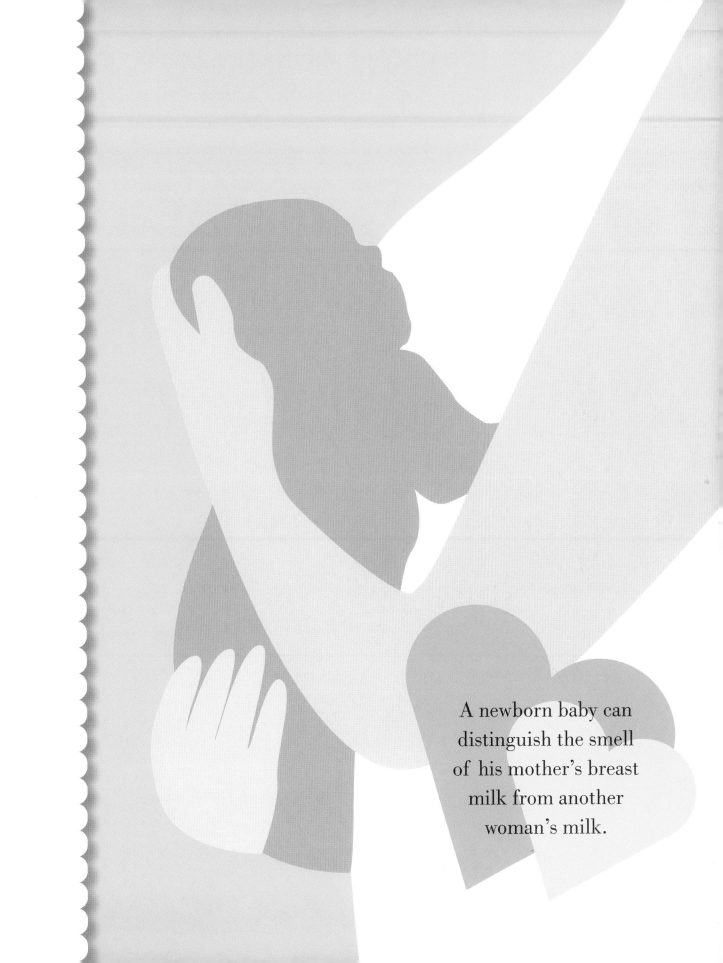

A newborn baby can distinguish the smell of his mother's breast milk from another woman's milk.

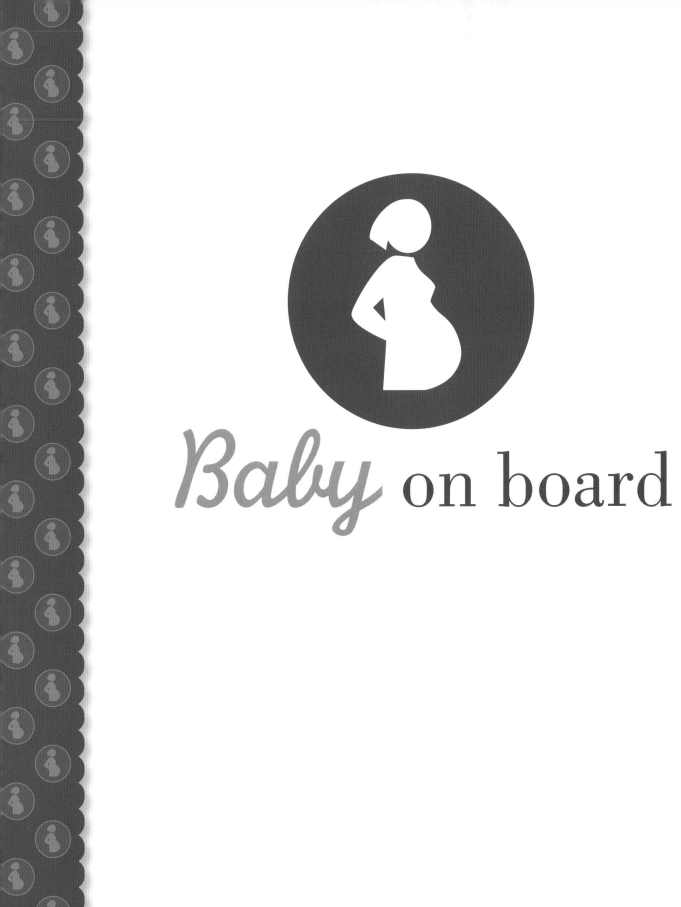

Baby on board

The first trimester
New *beginnings*

From that exhilarating moment when you read your positive pregnancy test, to the 13th week of pregnancy, your first trimester is a period of astonishing physical and emotional change. Your baby will grow from a single, microscopic cell into a tiny human being with eyes, nose, ears, mouth, and moving limbs, while your body starts to change to accommodate his needs and support his development. Expect your emotions to wobble and energy levels to fluctuate as your pregnancy hormones kick into action—you may feel everything from exhaustion and anxiety to excitement and elation over the coming weeks.

Congratulations, you are going to be a mom!

By the end of the first month, your baby is about the size of a grain of rice.

YOUR BABY'S HEART begins to beat as early as 22 days after fertilization—before you might know you are pregnant.

Some women experience a shortness of breath known as "air hunger" when they first become pregnant.

Until eight weeks your baby will have a tail that is about one-sixth of his length. It will eventually recede to form his tailbone.

About 20 percent of women will experience "implantation bleeding," when the fertilized egg implants in the uterus.

Your baby's brain waves can be recorded just six weeks after conception.

JEANS FEELING TIGHT? At six weeks your uterus has already expanded from the size of a plum to the size of a small orange.

By ten weeks, almost all of your baby's organs will be formed and some are already functioning.

By 11 weeks, your growing baby has 20 tooth buds in place, and soft nails start to form on his fingers and toes.

Your baby has his own unique fingerprints at 13 weeks.

The average woman (and we're all different) gains about 1–4½lb (500g to 2kg) in the first trimester, and about 1 lb (500g) a week thereafter.

The rate of twin pregnancies in some African countries, such as Nigeria, can be as high as 1 in 25. Whereas China has the lowest rate of twin births—1 in 300—in the world.

When sperm meets *egg*

The complex process of fertilization, when sperm and egg meet and fuse, is a carefully choreographed chain of events, each part crucial to the successful outcome of a viable pregnancy.

What's happening in the woman?

At birth, girls are born with their full quota of egg cells, about one to two million. From puberty through to menopause, the monthly menstrual cycle matures one or more eggs in response to follicle stimulating hormone, and builds up the uterine lining in preparation for a possible pregnancy. Midway through the cycle, a surge in luteinizing hormone triggers the release of the mature egg, which bursts out of the ovary some 35–42 hours later and into the fallopian tube, ready to greet the sperm. It will survive, unfertilized, for 24 hours.

What's happening in the man?

Men produce sperm throughout their lives from puberty, at a rate of around 1,500 sperm a second, and will release somewhere in the region of 180–400 million sperm per ejaculate: anything below 20 million sperm per milliliter is considered below par! Produced in the testes under the influence of testosterone and follicle stimulating hormone, a healthy sperm consists of an ovoid head, a neck, and a long tail with fibers that help to propel it along the female reproductive tract. During ejaculation, fluid from the male sex glands combines with the sperm to form semen, which is deposited close to the cervix, and the incredible race to penetrate the egg begins. This really is survival of the fittest, though, since each step of the journey is fraught with obstacles, and only one sperm will make it all the way.

An egg is the largest cell in a woman's body, measuring around 200 microns in diameter. By contrast a sperm is the smallest cell in a man's body, clocking in at just 2.5–3.5 microns across.

Sperm race

Right after ejaculation, semen coagulates to stop individual sperm from drifting off in the wrong direction—any that do lose their way perish in the acidic environment of the vagina. Within 5–40 minutes it re-liquefies and the sperm continue their journey through to the cervical canal, traveling $\frac{1}{16}$–$\frac{1}{8}$in (2–3 mm) per minute. At the fertile point of the menstrual cycle, cervical mucus becomes thin and watery to better enable the sperm to pass through the cervix. However, it's an uphill struggle and millions of sperm are lost along the way. Only around 100,000 enter the uterus (womb), and only 200–300 of those reach the correct fallopian tube; even then most drop away, and only a final few make it to the end of the tube to reach the waiting egg.

Final destination

Those sperm that finally reach their goal engulf the egg, sticking to its surface and releasing enzymes that, in combination, begin a chemical chain reaction that allows the egg's surface to be penetrated. While this may be a team effort, only one sperm will succeed in getting through, after which the egg undergoes an instant chemical reaction to prevent any other sperm from entering.

Two become one

The chromosomes of the egg and sperm that carry the genetic code fuse, and the sex of the baby is determined at that moment. The fertilized egg then gradually advances along the fallopian tube toward the uterus, undergoing a process of rapid cell division—starting as a single cell called a zygote, it eventually forms a mass of around 100 cells known as a blastocyst, which enters the uterus about six days after fertilization. The blastocyst burrows deeply into the thickened endometrial layer of the uterus; the inner cell mass will become the embryo, while the cells of its outer layer will become the placenta. The start of your pregnancy journey has begun!

The first day of *your new life*

You're pregnant, congratulations! You might be feeling a mixture of delight, excitement, and relief along with a little trepidation, ambivalence, and disbelief. The positive test result will change your life forever. Are you ready for what lies ahead?

It's natural to feel as anxious as you are excited, even if pregnancy is just what you were planning. And some days you may feel worried in the morning but by the afternoon you're delighted and ready to shout the news out to the world. All these feelings are totally normal as you adjust to the news and what it means for your future.

Looking ahead Now is not a time for rewinding through the past few days or weeks to wonder whether anything you've done could have affected your developing baby. What's important now is to take a fresh look at your life and lifestyle, and make positive changes for the future.

Celebrating this special time There has never been a safer time to have a baby, thanks, in part, to improving health care and prenatal care. Enjoy your pregnancy; you're doing the most magical of things—growing a baby.

Keeping mum Who to tell and when is a thought that'll be ever present for the next few weeks or so. You might be bursting to share the news but if it's not that long since your last period, then it's a good idea to wait until your next period is a no-show or to ask for a confirmatory test with your doctor. Many expectant parents wait until after the first ultrasound scan, between 10 and 12 weeks, but you should do whatever you feel is right for the two of you.

The trip of a lifetime You're about to take the first steps on the universal journey of parenthood. The next nine months will speed by in a flash, but the fun really starts when you get to meet your baby. In the meantime, build confidence in yourself and your partner by researching relevant issues and discussing and deciding together how you'd like things to pan out. There's one thing that's for sure, it's going to be one heck of a ride!

REALITY **CHECK**

How are you feeling?
You and your partner's emotions may be all over the place while you're adjusting to the news. Join the club if any or all of these fit your mood in a typical day: joyful, surprised, feeling isolated, lack of maternal/paternal instinct, anxiety about the birth, "I'm not ready," and disbelief. You're about to start an incredible journey, so give yourself time to adjust to the idea of family life. And relish your current freedom while you can.

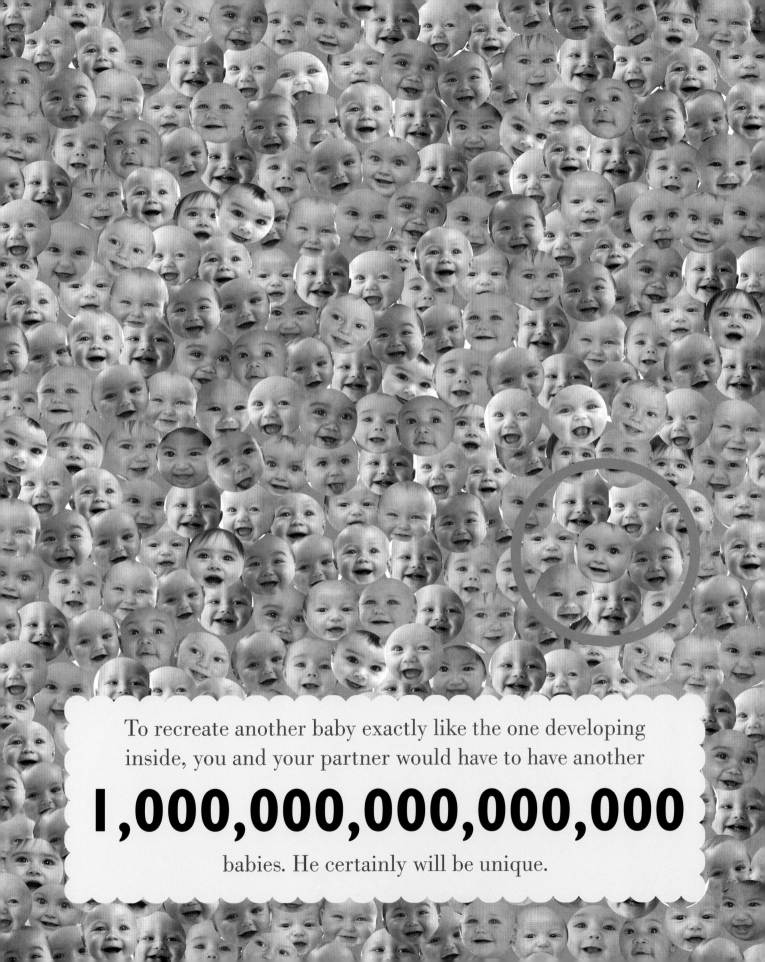

To recreate another baby exactly like the one developing inside, you and your partner would have to have another

1,000,000,000,000,000

babies. He certainly will be unique.

A new life *begins*

Your baby started off as a single, tiny cell, packed with potential.
This lone cell undergoes an incredible, intricate process of
multiplication until you have a baby made of trillions of cells.

Your baby's development is a complicated process, and yet her entire being derives from a single microscopic, three-layered ball of cells. The first stage of her development is when these cells differentiate and specialize, during which time your baby is referred to as an embryo. Once she has been developing for eight weeks, and for the rest of your pregnancy, she will be termed a fetus. By the end of the first trimester your baby has a human face and resembles a tiny person, with most of her body systems in place. She grows rapidly in the second trimester, and in the third her body fine-tunes itself ready to enter the world.

Officially, your baby's development is dated according to her "gestational" age. So when doctors talk about how many weeks pregnant you are, they are counting your pregnancy not from conception, but from the first day of your last period. So, when you are officially 12 weeks pregnant, your baby will have only been developing for ten weeks.

From one cell to over...
1,000,000,000,000
...in just nine months

August

Sun	Mon	Tue	Wed	Thu	Fri	Sat
29	30	31	1	2	3	4
5	6	7	8	9	10	11
12	13	14	15	16	17	18
19	20	21	22	23	24	25
26	27	28	29	30	31	

Journey to the uterus
Within 24 hours, the fertilized egg divides in two, then continues to split until a 100-celled ball (blastocyst) enters your uterus about **six days later**. Its inner layer of cells will form the embryo, while the outer layer burrows into the uterus lining. A placenta will develop from this outer layer of cells, but in the meantime the embryo is nourished from a yolk sac in the cavity.

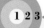

Laying the foundations

At week five of pregnancy, this tiny ball (now called an embryo) divides into three layers. Each layer gives rise to different parts of your baby's body. Her brain, spinal cord, skin, nervous system, eyes, ears, and connective tissues will be molded from the top layer. The middle layer will give your baby her heart, bones, muscles, and much of her reproductive system. The inner layer creates her lungs, bladder, and intestines.

Full speed ahead

By week six, your baby's body shape is forming. She is 1/16in (4mm) long and curves gently in a "C" shape, with a head and tail-end. Her simple heart pumps and arm and leg buds sprout from her body. Dotlike eyes form and on either side of her head tiny pits appear, from which ears will develop. **By week eight**, she is the size of a raspberry, her "tail" begins to disappear, her limbs lengthen, and little webbed fingers and toes start to appear.

Body systems are go

Between weeks 6 and 10, work on all your baby's major organs is in full swing. Cells in her body constantly divide and specialize into different roles. The first system to function is her cardiovascular system—vital so her heart can pump life-giving nutrients around her body to support her growth. This system constantly adapts and matures as she develops.

September

Sun	Mon	Tue	Wed	Thu	Fri	Sat
						1
2	3	4	5	6	7	8
9	10	11	12	13	14	15
16	17	18	19	20	21	22
23	24	25	26	27	28	29
30						

October

Sun	Mon	Tue	Wed	Thu	Fri	Sat
	1	2	3	4	5	6
7	8	9	10	11	12	13
14	15	16	17	18	19	20
21	22	23	24	25	26	27
28	29	30	31			

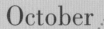

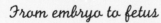

From embryo to fetus

Congratulations! **After eight frenetic weeks** of rapidly dividing, specializing, and remodeling itself, the embryo has graduated to become a fully fledged fetus. At about 1 in (3 cm) long she looks more like a human now as her face is taking shape. Her eyes are not yet covered by an eyelid, and she has a mouth and tongue.

And ready to grow...

At 12 weeks your baby is fully formed although only the size of a plum. She has reflexes and may respond to gentle pressure on your tummy. She may suck her thumb, swallow amniotic fluid, and pass urine. Your baby has made it through the most vulnerable stages of her development and from here on her body must grow and mature so that when birth comes she is ready for the world.

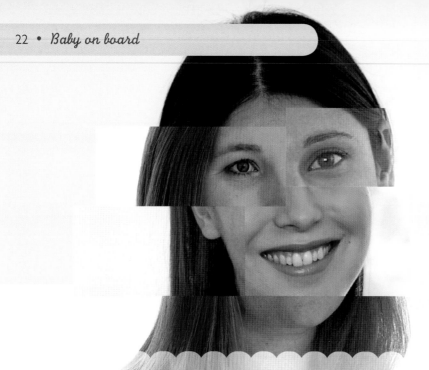

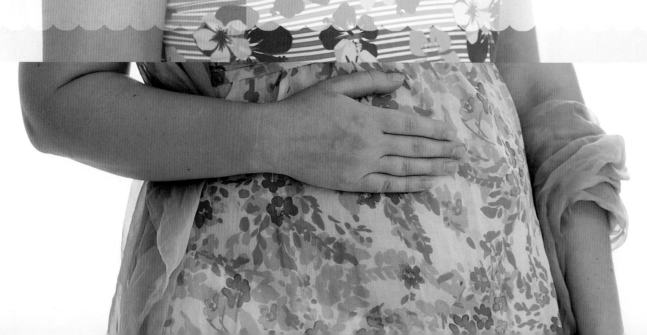

Not quite *yourself?*

You may feel different when you're pregnant—even before a test reads positive. If you suddenly cannot stand the taste of your regular coffee, or your partner's scent makes you queasy, this might be a clue that changes are already underway.

Metallic mouth

An unpleasant metallic taste in the mouth, known as dysgeusia, can be caused by higher estrogen levels, as well as the effects of water retention on your taste buds. Weirdly, eating sweet foods can exacerbate the mineral taste in your mouth, but brushing your teeth and tongue with mint toothpaste can help, as can eating acidic foods or sprinkling vinegar on your salad or french fries.

Strange tastes

Does your food need more salt, or taste bitter? Higher estrogen levels can have a real effect on your sense of taste: reduced sensitivity to saltiness and increased sensitivity to bitter food is common (see pages 38–39). Many women naturally have a distaste for coffee and alcohol in the first trimester, but this is probably a good thing.

Motion commotion

If you are prone to motion sickness, unfortunately this may be more acute when pregnant and you are more likely to experience morning sickness. Low blood-sugar levels seem to trigger nausea, so eat regular meals and snacks, particularly before a long trip or commute. Travel wristbands may help since they press on an acupressure spot at the inner wrist. For general tips on beating nausea, see right.

Stand well back

Your breasts are likely to feel supersensitive—pity the partner or toddler who accidentally brushes your chest. This is a result of your breasts swelling in preparation for breast-feeding. Wearing a supportive bra without an underwire should help them feel more comfortable.

What's that smell?

Your sense of smell is intertwined with your sense of taste and is also affected by your estrogen levels. Many pregnant women report heightened sensitivity to smell: avid gardeners may find the scent of certain plants intolerable and vintage fiends may find the smell of second-hand shops revolting. Other women report "phantom" smells, or notice ones from a long distance away. Try masking nauseating scents with refreshing lemon: place two drops of essential oil of lemon on a cloth and sniff when you need to.

Drooling like a baby

Extra saliva is a classic symptom of early pregnancy, and may be caused by the increased levels of human chorionic gonadotrophin, the hormone that sustains pregnancy. This is at its peak in the first 8 to 11 weeks, but should calm down after that. Chew gum, drink plenty of water, and eat little and often to make yourself feel more comfortable.

Need a quick nap?

Pregnancy fatigue can be especially overwhelming at this early stage. It's caused by increased progesterone and your body working hard to grow a new life. In preparation for the new baby your body needs to increase its blood volume and is busy consuming more oxygen—this is tiring work! Take every opportunity for a daytime nap, take it easy when you get home from work, and ease up on your social calendar.

BEAT THE **SICKNESS**

Nibble an oat or ginger cookie before you get out of bed in the morning.

Eat oats for breakfast in oatmeal, granola, muesli, smoothies, or pancakes. Their slow-release energy boosts energy levels, builds stamina, and staves off nausea.

Eat little and often to stabilize your blood sugar levels. Carbohydrates, such as pasta, bread, and rice, can help so include them in your meals.

Try ginger in tea, smoothies, juices, or capsules to beat nausea. It encourages good digestion, and counters constipation and indigestion.

Drink diluted lemon juice to encourage your appetite.

Get plenty of fresh air since stale air can make you feel tired and queasy.

Decisions
decisions...

Once the news has sunk in, you'll find yourself reassessing certain aspects of life that once seemed set in stone. Don't panic—a calm, rational look at your options will reassure, and may even open doors.

Many parents-to-be don't announce news of pregnancy until the second trimester when the risk of miscarriage declines. However, it is nice to share your excitement with a few select loved ones. This can be tricky to arrange—it may not be possible to tell both sets of your parents together, but will one feel insulted if the other finds out first? If you tell one friend, must you then tell another? Don't let this wonderful moment be clouded by emotional politics—be positive in your decisions and don't bow to any pressure. It is your baby, and your choice.

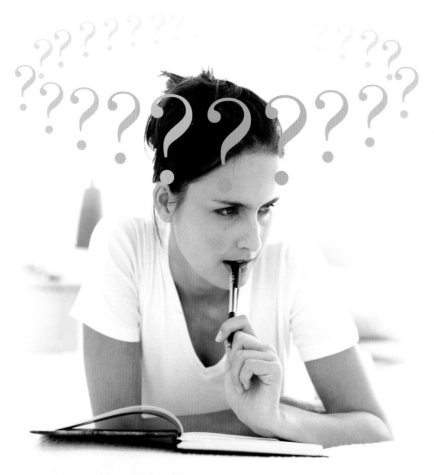

I'm worrying about money already.

Uncertainty can lead to anxiety and even depression, so make financial plans now. First figure out your incomings and outgoings, then find out what maternity benefits, tax credits, and time off you are entitled to. Look into child-care costs, and the pros and cons of flexible or part-time work.

Does my career have to be put on hold?

Not necessarily, but many women find that pregnancy forces them to rethink their working lives in a more family-friendly way. This doesn't have to be a detriment to a career, and freelance or part-time work can open up new and unexpected opportunities.

The trip to work seems exhausting.

Traveling in the first 12 weeks can feel overwhelming while

❁ Try to see your pregnancy as a liberating time when you can throw everything up in the air and make exciting decisions about your future.

your body is working so hard at growing a baby. Could you arrange to work more flexibly to avoid rush hour? Even though no belly bump will be evident, most people will offer you a seat if asked—don't hold back, this is not a time to struggle.

Will I turn into my mother?

Becoming a parent forces you to look at how you were parented and make choices about which elements of your childhoods to replicate, let go, or rework. The process starts in pregnancy, when families throw all sorts of advice your way. You choose how much to take on, don't feel obliged to accept their views as your own. Remember it is your baby!

Our relationship feels different.

It's bound to—your lives are linked together forever as a result of your pregnancy, and now there are three people in the relationship. Many parents-to-be feel closer, but some can feel a little trapped. Make sure you talk openly about any anxieties— good communication is vital and you may find that your partner is experiencing similar worries.

My apartment is tiny. How will we all fit in?

Be reassured that babies are tiny and don't need quite as much paraphernalia as magazines suggest. Be organized and figure out what you'll need for just the first three months, then you can make an informed decision on what more to get. What can you borrow from friends or family? Take advice from friends who are parents whose opinion you trust.

❁ Keep things in perspective: you and your baby have to come first now, and the rest of life will have to adapt to accommodate that.

Month 2

weeks 5–8

All about you

Ready to make milk
Your breasts are already gearing up for breast-feeding, adding milk glands and fat layers, and getting larger as a result. These changes and pregnancy hormones can cause breast tenderness—seasoned moms often recognize this as the first sign of pregnancy.

Room for baby
Your uterus will expand from the size of a walnut to a large orange over this period, and you may feel an unusual stretching sensation. Don't be alarmed, your baby's home is being prepared.

Super stretchy
Levels of the hormone relaxin rise early on in pregnancy, released first by the corpus luteum and later by the placenta. With its almost self-explanatory name, relaxin softens ligaments, ultimately to widen your pelvis for birth; but, in the meantime, it makes joints more lax. So, your yoga poses and stretches may improve with this new-found flexibility, but just be aware that the downside can be backaches and hypermobile joints.

Keep taking folic acid
It's essential in the early months for the healthy development of your baby's brain, spinal cord, and nervous system.

Crazy cravings
You may have intense cravings, or find overnight that you can't stomach certain foods. Theories as to why range from the effects of hormones to your body sensing the need for specific nutrients.

Feeling a little delicate
Soaring progesterone levels relax blood vessels so they can manage the extra blood flow. This relaxes the digestive tract, too, and, together with an enhanced sense of smell and extra stomach acid, can cause nausea; this usually falls away in the second trimester.

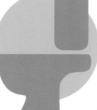

Up and down

Hormonal surges in early pregnancy can have dramatic effects on mood, and you and your partner may need to adapt your mindset to accommodate unpredictable mood swings, and try to avoid triggers. Hormones aside, this time is intense for you both as you mentally adjust to the idea of having a baby. You may find excitement mingling with feelings of guilt over misgivings. Ambivalence is normal as you process this monumental life change.

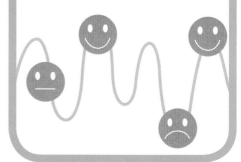

Your metabolic rate increases by 10 to 25 percent during pregnancy to support the increased activity of your organs.

 At week 8 your baby measures about **⅔in** (1.6 cm) crown to rump.

0 (cm)   **10**   **20**

Your growing baby

* Major eye structures are already forming, and your baby will develop eyelids by the end of eight weeks. His eyelids remain fused until much later in pregnancy.

* Arm and leg buds appear early in pregnancy, followed by little webbed fingers and toes. By the end of this month, his arms will bend at the wrist and the elbow.

* Tooth buds are forming, and a tongue is evident. Rudimentary taste buds will be working soon, and he'll taste what you eat!

* The central nervous system, which links your baby's muscles to his brain, is developing, and basic reflexes are in place.

* Muscle and bone tissue are building up, and will continue to develop throughout pregnancy.

* At the end of two months, your baby's heart will be fully developed and beating 150 times every minute (about twice that of an adult).

* The liver is beginning to produce red blood cells, which will carry oxygen in his body, and small veins are already evident beneath his skin.

* At eight weeks, your baby is officially known as a fetus, with refined facial features, distinct limbs, hands and feet, as well as fingers and toes.

1st week

Your baby undergoes dramatic changes in these first weeks. From a seed-sized bundle of cells, growth is rapid, and by eight weeks he's becoming recognizably human.

| Poppy seed | Apple seed | Pea | Blueberry | Raspberry |

This month, think about...

Looking ahead
It's not too early to think about where you might want to give birth. Your first appointment is an opportunity to discuss your options and find out what is, and isn't, available. Thinking about this now doesn't mean you can't change your mind later on.

The good of the group
Have you considered childbirth classes? Childbirth classes will fill up early on, so you may need to reserve a spot now.

Up for a scan?
Thought about which scans you might want? There are fixed time periods for scans and the first ones are imminent. Some are routinely offered, but others vary between practices—your doctor will discuss details and availability. You may be tempted by a 3D or video scan, which you'll need to arrange with your doctor.

30   40   50

Pregnancy *Superfoods*

There has never been a better time than now to switch to eating healthier foods—to provide both the energy you need for the extra demands of pregnancy and the right blend of baby-building ingredients. In your second and third trimesters, you will need to eat 300 extra calories each day—but try to make sure your choices count nutritionally.

Avocado

These non-fruity pears pack a healthy nutrient punch: with vitamins C and B6, good for your baby's tissue and brain growth; potassium, which helps to regulate your fluid balance; and folate, the naturally occurring form of folic acid, vital for your baby's developing nervous system. Delicious sliced into a salad, or mashed for an appetizing topping on a whole-grain slice. Don't go crazy, though, as avocados are high in fat, too.

Broccoli

All types of broccoli contain carotenoids—antioxidants that are good for your baby's eyesight, and potassium, which regulates blood pressure as well as fluid balance. Broccoli also contains vitamins A and C, which transfer to your baby. Try it steamed, added to a stir-fry, or in soup.

Cheese

Pasteurized hard and soft cheeses contain calcium, phosphorus, and magnesium that strengthen both your bones and your baby's. Since cheese is fairly high in fat, eat small amounts or grate it over dishes. Avoid any homemade or artisanal cheeses that aren't labeled "pasteurized."

Eggs

An easy option for a quick meal any time of day, eggs are a good source of protein and contain essential amino acids, vitamins, and minerals; though they need to be cooked well. Eggs are rich in the mineral choline—crucial for your baby's brain development and improves your memory, too.

Bananas

Rich in potassium, bananas are good for reducing fluid retention and also contain the amino acid tryptophan, which promotes good sleep. Slice onto cereal for breakfast, whizz into smoothies, or enjoy solo as a perfectly portable energy-boosting snack.

Sweet potato

Along with folate, fiber, and potassium, sweet potatoes also contain vitamin C, which helps to boost your baby's immunity and strengthen her bones, teeth, and blood vessels. You can bake a sweet potato, mash it, or cut it into wedges to go with grilled cheese, fish, or meat.

Whole-grain foods

Oats, whole-wheat bread and pasta, rye bread, brown rice, quinoa, and other whole-grain foods contain more nutrients and fiber (which helps prevent constipation) than processed grains. Try oatmeal or muesli in the morning, and whole-wheat pasta for dinner.

Salmon

In addition to protein and B vitamins, salmon contains the omega-3 fats that promote healthy brain growth and the development of your baby's vision. Grill a quick-cooking salmon steak to go with a salad, or use canned salmon for a sandwich or to make fish cakes.

Beef

Lean cuts of quality beef give you an iron boost, so if you are feeling tired, a steak might pep you up. Iron aids the transfer of oxygen to your baby, wards off anemia, and can prevent premature delivery. Beef also contains easily absorbable forms of cell-building protein, zinc, and B vitamins.

Berries

As well as being an excellent source of vitamin C, berries are rich in antioxidants that help to fight free radicals and prevent cell damage. Snack or breakfast on fresh blueberries, blackberries, raspberries, and strawberries, or add frozen or fresh berries to smoothies, yogurt, and porridge.

I need a drink

Your changing body and your growing baby both need you to be hydrated. So, what's best to drink and what, if anything, should you avoid?

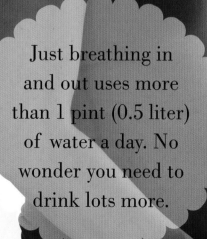

From week six or seven of your first trimester, your blood volume increases so that you can transport nutrients around your body and to your developing baby, and carry waste products away from your baby. To do this efficiently, you need more hydration, which basically equals water. Water is also required to manufacture and renew the amniotic fluid that bathes your baby during pregnancy. What's more, hydration is good for you too: supporting kidney and liver function, keeping your brain alert, helping prevent constipation, and flushing out bacteria that trigger pregnancy urinary-tract infections. And strange as it sounds, drinking plenty of water combats water retention. Keep a bottle of water handy to sip throughout the day—by the time you're thirsty you're already dehydrated.

How much to drink

Some 19 percent of your daily hydration comes from food, so you have to drink 81 percent in liquid form. Recommended daily intake varies from country to country, and there's no agreed US level; though 8 glasses (64floz) daily. is usually recommended for women. Fluid requirements during pregnancy are a tad higher—about 1fl oz (30ml) extra daily.

> Just breathing in and out uses more than 1 pint (0.5 liter) of water a day. No wonder you need to drink lots more.

Best beverages

Water is healthiest but if you prefer something zingier, add a squeeze of lemon or lime, or some fruit juice. Milk is great for calcium, vitamins A and D, and lean protein, and a small glass of fruit juice or smoothie counts as one of your daily portions of fruit and vegetables.

Avoid alcoholic beverages

It's not safe to have any amount of alcohol in your system while you're pregnant. Alcohol has been linked to preventable birth defects and mental retardation, and it increases the risk of miscarriage, low birthweight, and stillbirth. If you're going out socially, sip soda or a glass of water, or ask for a virgin cocktail.

REALITY **CHECK**

Caffeine calculations

Now is the time to revisit your caffeine intake—but this doesn't mean an end to your morning latte or an afternoon mugful. A sensible limit is 200 mg a day; check the caffeine-o-meter (right). Caffeine can interfere with iron and folic acid absorption, and has been associated with lower birth-weight babies. And, a little warning, decaffeinated drinks do contain caffeine, just tinier amounts. The bad news is that chocolate does contain caffeine; the good news is you'd have to eat over eight milk chocolate bars before hitting the limit.

Caffeine is a mild diuretic, which eliminates water and promotes dehydration.

Caffeine-o-meter

Can of cola
35 mg

Mug of tea
75 mg

Green tea
30 mg

Mug of filtered coffee
140 mg

Mug of filter coffee, decaf
10 mg

Mug of instant coffee
100 mg

Single espresso
50–300 mg

Regular latte
40–75 mg

Plain chocolate (2 oz/50 g)
50 mg

Milk chocolate (2 oz/50 g)
25 mg

Does *age* matter?

The average age for a first-time mother is rising with each generation. If you are over 35, you may be labeled an "older mother" but you are not alone.

Seeing the words "**elderly primigravida**" in your medical chart can be somewhat alarming. Rather than being some kind of insult, it's simply med-speak for a woman of **35 years or older who is pregnant for the first time**. However, if you fall into this category, this tag can be a disheartening reaffirmation of the much-repeated notion that older mothers are "at risk." Why can't you just be a normal mom-to-be? Take heart, there are many things to celebrate about being an older mother. Women in their 30s and early 40s may well have a **physical and psychological advantage** over younger women. They are often better at taking care of themselves and lead a **healthier lifestyle**, as well as being more **highly educated** and **financially secure**. Furthermore, age usually brings increased **self-confidence** and **self-esteem**, which can have a positive effect on pregnancy and parenthood.

You are in good company: statistics show a marked trend in recent years toward women **delaying parenthood until their thirties**, with the 35–39-year age bracket seeing the biggest rise. Doctors view older mothers as having more **risks** in pregnancy: a higher risk of developing complications, such as gestational diabetes, high blood pressure, a low-lying placenta, and having a premature birth. Also, older moms are more likely to have to undergo invasive tests to check for genetic abnormalities. The flip side to these medical risks is that you will have a higher level of doctor care and can be reassured by the **extra monitoring** of your baby. Your pregnancy is as exciting as anyone else's, so enjoy it to the fullest.

Did you know?

✳ **Older women tend to have a more positive body image—they are often healthier and stronger, and so deal better with the natural changes pregnancy brings to the body.**

Older mothers have usually achieved more personal goals, so are less likely to feel they are "missing out" by focusing solely on family.

✳ **Children with older mothers often develop a broader vocabulary from a young age, are brighter, and achieve higher scores in IQ tests.**

✳ More years on the clock means a greater pool of life skills and experience to rely on when navigating pregnancy and parenthood; it may also mean a wider circle of friends and family to draw on for support.

✳ *One study found that new mothers over 40 are four times more likely to live to be 100 years old than younger mothers.*

✳ A healthy lifestyle and good nutrition can help counteract fatigue during pregnancy, so, contrary to popular belief, older mothers may not find pregnancy more tiring.

Month 3

All about you

Is that a baby in there?
Your uterus will soon be the size of a small melon and extend above your pelvic bone. Your waistline may expand slightly, and very slender moms-to-be may begin to "show."

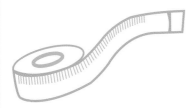

Your growing uterus
The expansion of your uterus is supported by the increased blood supply to the pelvic area. By 12 weeks, this accounts for up to a quarter of the total blood volume.

An incredible organ
By the end of this month, your placenta is structurally complete and takes over the job of nurturing your baby from the yolk sac. This complex organ is his life-support system now, nourishing him and protecting him from harmful substances and infections.

Extra iron, please
Iron supports the oxygen-carrying capacity of your red blood cells, and you need almost double the amount now. Supplements aren't needed unless advised, but eat iron-rich foods daily.

Take a deep breath
Your chest actually expands now to increase your lung capacity, allowing you to breathe deeply to take in more oxygen. As breathing deepens and quickens, it's normal to feel breathless and light-headed at times.

O_2

How much?

You may gasp when you see estimates of the cost of raising a child, but there are ways to minimize the expense. Compiling a spreadsheet of necessary items and whether you can borrow rather than buy highlights potential savings. Can you minimize future child-care costs too—share a nanny, or call on willing and able family members?

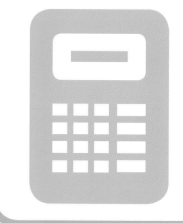

By 8–14 weeks, your blood volume has increased by 10 to 15 percent.

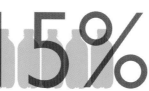

15%

 At week 8

 By the end of this month, your baby measures **2 in** (5 cm) crown to rump.

By 12 weeks
Your baby will be the size of a plum.

> **At around 12 weeks,** your first ultrasound provides the first glimpse of your tiny baby. Prepare to be amazed!

Your growing baby

* Your amazing baby can already curl his toes and open and close his fingers. You may be able to see these movements at your first ultrasound.

* His skeleton is complete, and is formed mostly of cartilage (rather than bone), which makes him flexible enough to negotiate the birth canal. His bones will begin to harden over the coming months and after the birth.

* Internal organs are formed by the end of nine weeks, and they'll continue to mature throughout pregnancy.

* Your baby is becoming increasingly active, and he'll raise his arms, touch his face, rotate in his comfortable new home, and even yawn and hiccup.

* There is a wonderfully light peach fuzz over his body, which protects him from the amniotic fluid and keeps him warm until he begins to lay down fat.

* His miniature heart has four functioning chambers (just like yours) and it's beating strongly.

* Reflexes are now developing, and your baby may respond when you press firmly on your belly.

This month, think about...

Spreading the news
If you haven't already done so, have you thought about when to spread the happy news? For many, the perfect moment is after the first scan, when it all seems much more real.

Pregnancy and work
When will you tell colleagues? While there are no rules, doing it earlier means you can discuss plans, and your boss will appreciate knowing about doctor appointments.

Squeeze and hold
Pelvic muscles stretch from 12 weeks, so starting Kegel exercises now helps them deal better in late pregnancy, and avoids a leaky bladder later on.

Breast care
Your breasts enlarge early on, which means you need a well-fitted, supportive maternity bra. Look out for one with wide straps and support under and at the sides of your breasts.

Fit and *well*

Jumping on a treadmill may be furthest from your
mind when you 're struggling to cope with nausea and fatigue,
but keeping in shape now has some real benefits later on.

Can I workout at the gym? * *Is it ok to run?* * *Can I ride my bike?*

Why is it so important?

Regular, gentle exercise keeps you
supple, toning muscles and helping
your body deal better with pregnancy
aches and pains. Minor complaints
such as constipation and swelling can
be reduced, or even eliminated, with
regular activity, which keeps the
bowels and circulation moving.

Prepare for labor

Moderate aerobic workouts increase
your stamina and will help make your
labor more efficient—and shorter.
Being in good shape will also speed
up your postpartum recovery and help
you deal with the
challenging early
weeks with a
newborn.

What a lift

It's common to feel
drained in pregnancy, but staying
active boosts flagging energy levels.
Keeping fit increases cardiovascular
efficiency and strengthens muscles,
which in turn means you expend less
energy overall—simple! In addition,
exercising also releases a rush of
endorphins, giving you a natural high.

How relaxing!

Exercise has some more subtle effects
too. It increases levels of the mood-
enhancing brain chemical serotonin,
and studies show that women who
stay active in pregnancy experience
less insomnia, stress, and
depression. It's easy to see
the rolling effects—activity

leads to better sleep; feeling rested
reduces anxiety; and the risk factors
for depression are reduced.

Good for baby, too

Exercising in pregnancy may even
give your baby a healthy head start.
A 2010 New Zealand study found that
pregnant women who did moderate
aerobic exercise had babies with a
slightly lower birthweight, which
could mean fewer health risks ahead.
Another study found that babies born
to moms who exercised had healthier
heart rates, suggesting that a
cardiovascular workout for mom
exercised the baby's heart, too!

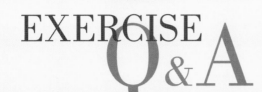

Should I start yoga?

EXERCISE Q&A

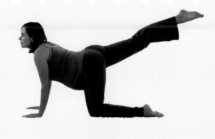

Is bicycling off the agenda?

Even if you're a proficient cyclist, put away your bike for the rest of your pregnancy. As your belly grows, your center of gravity changes, making falls more likely. Play it safe and move to a stationary bike instead.

Can I begin exercising now?

A vow to get more fit now is a good thing, but be realistic and stick to gentle exercise that won't push you past your limits, such as walking, yoga, or swimming—all of which are ideal for pregnancy.

How will I know if I'm overdoing it?

A good indication that you are pushing yourself too hard is if you cannot keep talking easily while exercising. So, if that's the case, slow it down.

Can I continue running?

While this isn't the time to take up jogging, if you're a seasoned runner and have a straightforward pregnancy, it's generally considered safe. Avoid running in hot conditions, and perhaps stick to a moderate distance and speed.

Is yoga really that helpful?

Yes, it honestly does have fantastic benefits. Aside from from toning and strengthening muscles, its holistic approach and focus on breathing give you the know-how to relax and can have a real impact on how you deal with contractions in labor.

What about Kegel exercises?

Strengthening the sling of muscles that form your pelvic floor helps you avoid stress incontinence after the birth. Start these now (see page 160) to reap the rewards after the birth.

SENSE AND SENSIBILITY

Sensible precautions ensure safe exercise for you and your baby. The pregnancy hormone relaxin softens ligaments, which can make you feel more flexible than you are, so don't overstretch, and make sure to warm up and cool down. Avoid short bursts of high-intensity exercise, don't get too breathless, and stay hydrated. Some activities are best avoided, such as horseback riding and skiing where there's a risk of falling, as well as lifting heavy weights, or twisting or jerky moves. Listen to your body: don't push yourself and stop if you experience pain or strain.

Simply being pregnant engages you in low level aerobic exercise since your heart rate increases by up to 20 percent.

What's with the *cravings?*

You are what you eat—but what does that mean when suddenly you find yourself putting ketchup on bananas?

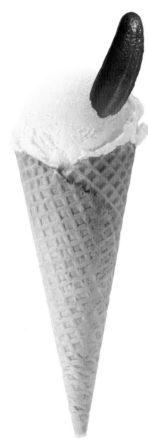

In soap operas, a strange craving for ice cream and pickles is a sure sign of a pregnancy in the story line, and we have all heard of a friend who suddenly wanted to eat lots of red meat, or completely avoided their regular coffee fix. In fact, at least 75 percent of pregnant women **crave specific foods** at some stage during their 40 weeks.

It might come as no surprise that the most popular craving is for sweet, fatty foods, such as chocolate or donuts, followed by salty snacks and spicy foods, but this does vary according to your background. In Tanzania, for example, meat is the number one pregnancy craving, with mangoes, yogurt, and oranges coming close behind, whereas Cambodian women crave significantly spicy and salty foods.

The flip side of cravings are **food aversions,** which can strike just as unexpectedly. The sudden and compulsive nature of a food craving or aversion can be very surprising; you simply must have that burned toast with lots of butter, no matter the time of day or night.

When do these curious likes and dislikes strike? Food cravings seem **more marked in first pregnancies** though researchers couldn't pinpoint a common time when they started for the women asked. However, 60 percent of food aversions **begin during the first trimester** when nausea kicks in, according to the journal *Appetite.* Aversions seem less troublesome after the first trimester, but cravings can continue throughout pregnancy. A study from the same journal also found that women consumed significantly more sweet food during the second trimester, while University of Connecticut researchers have tracked an increase in cravings for salty foods as the weeks progress.

So, what's going on? Some commentators say cravings demonstrate the **body's intuitive knowledge** of the nutrients it lacks. While this might be true for dairy cravings, given that the average woman gets only three-quarters of the calcium she needs, it can't be applied to salty snacks. Though we do need a little extra sodium as our blood volume increases, most of us already eat too much salt. There is no good evidence to support this theory.

Another theory suggests that food aversions are a built-in **protective mechanism** safeguarding mother and baby from environmental toxins. Witness the numbers of women who suddenly find the very thought of coffee nauseating, especially during the early weeks of pregnancy. Many toxic plants share its bitterness and pungency.

A more likely cause of both cravings and aversions is **hormonal change**. Researchers have tracked cravings in relation to levels of progesterone and prolactin, which can influence appetite. Hormonal changes have a sensitizing effect on our sense of smell and taste, and there seem to be strong links, too, with the texture of the foods craved. Ice is a popular pregnancy craving for the delicious crunch as much as its cooling and hydrating effects.

One study found that pregnant women who noticed a change in their sense of smell had substantially more cravings.

There's evidence that **cravings are influenced** by what we grow up thinking we should crave, such as fruit and dairy that traditional Ayurveda medicine considers cooling, or the popular clichés we see on television. Cravings can intensify during **periods of anxiety,** and pregnancy can be an unsettling time. It's tempting to turn to comfort foods, and many pregnant women express a longing for bland childhood favorites, such as grilled-cheese sandwiches, pudding, or buttered pasta. There may be value in this, since carbohydrates boost levels of the hormone serotonin, helping you feel relaxed.

The name pica derives from the Latin term for a magpie (*Pica pica*), the bird that grabs anything that takes its fancy.

But **cravings can go crazy.** Some pregnant women find themselves creeping downstairs at night to eat the scale from the inside of a tea kettle or sniffing shoe polish. This is **pica,** a craving for non-food items, most commonly soil, clay, and laundry starch. This pregnancy phenomenon is documented across cultures and as far back as the Greco-Roman era. In some traditions cravings are expected and even encouraged as a means of protection or to augur good fortune. In a study in 2000, Mexican mothers told of eating small blocks of holy clay stamped with the image of the Virgin of Guadalupe for blessings, and that resisting a craving could mean your baby is never satisfied ("born with its mouth open"), while satisfying your craving helps to create a happy ("cleansed") baby.

So, **should you resist** pregnancy cravings? If you're tempted to sniff car exhaust or nibble coal, yes, and maybe have a word with your doctor about whether you are lacking anything in your diet. But no data suggest that giving in to food cravings is bad for your baby. What you might want to do is think about substituting healthier choices, such as frozen yogurt instead of ice cream or popcorn for donuts; also eat **little and often** since low blood-sugar levels can trigger cravings. Eating more fish may help since the oil is thought to reduce cravings. If you're obsessing about chocolate, you might be lacking magnesium and would benefit from snacking on flax or sunflower seeds. Fatigue can intensify cravings, so make sure you get plenty of sleep at night and rest during the day and, above all, nurture yourself through this **strange and precious** stage of your life.

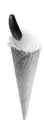

The second trimester
Time to *blossom*

The second trimester, running from 14 to 27 weeks, is often termed the "planning" or "golden" trimester—and with good reason. You may experience a period of renewed energy and comfort, and find that your excitement builds as you acclimatize to pregnancy and start to concentrate on preparing for your new arrival. With her organs and body systems in place, your baby will grow at a tremendous rate now, and so will your belly! This is a period when things will feel more settled, so make the most of it—spread the news, spend some quality time with your partner, and enjoy this special time in your life. For a few more months you can simply enjoy yourself.

It won't be long before you feel those first fluttering movements!

An increase in blood volume helps lend your skin that radiant pregnancy "glow."

By about 19 weeks, your baby will "practice" breathing movements, drawing amniotic fluid into her lungs and then "exhaling" it.

Your body temperature is slightly higher throughout pregnancy. You'll perspire more readily to get rid of the heat from you and your baby.

A 20-WEEK-OLD BABY is the weight and length of a banana.

Most moms-to-be feel their babies move for the first time (called "quickening") at about 20 weeks; it feels like a goldfish flipping or popcorn popping.

Around 15–18 weeks, your baby starts to develop a dark layer of very fine downy hair on her head, known as "lanugo," which is Latin for "wool." Within a few weeks, she'll be totally covered in the stuff.

At 24 weeks, your baby can tell the difference between Mom's and Dad's voices and will remember a piece of music she has heard frequently while in the uterus.

By 25 weeks, your heart and lungs are working up to 50 percent harder than before you were pregnant.

LANGUAGE ACQUISITION begins at about 25 weeks, as babies listen repeatedly to their mothers' intonation and learn the speech rhythms of their mother tongue.

Practicing your Kegel exercises for just five minutes, three times a day, can shorten the pushing stage of labor.

At 26 weeks, the height of the top of your uterus is approximately 10 in (26 cm).

A baby born at 26 weeks has an 80 percent chance of survival.

During the second trimester, your blood volume doubles.

Month 4

All about you

In the mood
Extra estrogen, and overactive mucous membranes, increase vaginal discharge, which should be colorless and odorless. This extra lubrication can make sex particularly pleasurable now!

What was that?
Your uterus sits about 2 in (5 cm) below your belly button now. Experienced moms may feel the first movements,; it may feel like a tiny fish is flapping around in there.

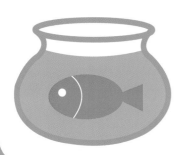

Raring to go
As your hormones stabilize, any nausea usually recedes and you'll feel on a more even keel and quite possibly brimming with energy.

Time to shine
Are you positively glowing? The effects of high progesterone levels and increased blood volume may be outwardly evident now as skin glows and hair is shiny and lush.

Tuning in
Studies show that babies move in response to sound as early as 16 weeks of pregnancy. As your voices become familiar to him, bonding can start. Instinctively you rub your belly, sing, and talk to him to let him know you're there, and he's comforted by that.

Your breasts are ahead of the game and may already have begun to manufacture colostrum, your baby's very "first" milk.

Your kidneys' filtering capacity has increased by up to 60 percent.

60%

 By the end of this month, your baby measures **4¾ in** (12 cm).

0 (cm)　　　　　　　　　10　　　　　　　　　20

By week 15
Your baby has his first growth spurt at around 15 weeks. He doubles in weight and grows inches longer. By the end of this month he will be the size of a large avocado.

Your growing baby

* The tiny bones in your baby's ears are in place by 16 weeks and he is capable now of hearing sounds within the uterus, which is alive with the sound of your heartbeat, blood flow, and digestion.

* Although his sucking reflexes are not yet fully developed, your baby's primitive "rooting reflex," which encourages him to open his mouth to search for your nipple at birth, is already well established by now.

* His neck begins to elongate as his chin is raised off his chest and he unfurls in his comfortable home.

* His kidneys are now producing urine, which is released into the amniotic fluid. This fluid provides him with a cushion, and gives him space to move; it is also important to help his lungs develop since it allows them to expand.

* He's starting to develop a dark layer of very fine, downy hair known as "lanugo" (Latin for "wool"), which insulates him and prevents him from becoming waterlogged.

* Although his eyes are closed, he will respond to bright light outside the uterus.

This month, think about...

● **A new wardrobe**
Since it gets harder to zip up, you'll need to invest in maternity items. A few basics can suffice, and be added to if needed.

● **Back care**
Watching your posture, doing a gentle exercise routine, and checking out appropriate back-strengthening exercises pays dividends later in pregnancy.

● **The birth**
Putting some thought into birth preferences now can help clarify what kind of birth you want, and whether you need to prepare, for example by arranging a birth preparation course, such as a hypnobirthing..

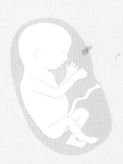

30   40   50

Your amazing *body*

During pregnancy, your body becomes a finely tuned baby-making machine, undergoing a host of invisible changes.

Exponential growth

Your uterus expands 1,000 times during pregnancy, from the size of a plum to the size of a watermelon. Its liquid capacity changes from holding ⅓fl oz (10ml) to holding more than 10½ pints (5 liters). Your uterus is protected by a plug of thick mucus that forms in the cervix—this seals the entrance to the uterus and prevents any bacteria from entering and potentially harming your baby.

Blood matters

From month four, your blood volume increases significantly to ensure an adequate supply to your uterus. Your blood vessels dilate so that the blood flows closer to the skin, giving you your pregnancy "glow." To keep the extra blood moving around, your heart will pump faster—7 more beats per minute in the early months and up to 15 extra beats later on.

Baby lifeline

You will grow a whole new organ—the placenta. It filters oxygen and nutrients to your baby as well as secreting the necessary hormones. It also transfers some of your immunities into your unborn baby. It is pretty substantial too—a full-term placenta will be about 6⅓–8in (16–20cm) in diameter and weigh about 17½oz (half a kilogram).

Deep breaths

Your lungs adapt to the extra demand for oxygen by increasing their capacity. Progesterone affects the way in which oxygen and carbon dioxide are absorbed into your bloodstream. What's more, you become more sensitive to levels of carbon dioxide, causing you to breathe more deeply.

Getting hot in here

Your body temperature is likely to be a little higher than normal during your pregnancy, this is due to increased levels of progesterone as well as an increase in your metabolism.

Baby brain

Your brain actually rewires itself during pregnancy, creating new connections that are thought to help you focus on your baby. While initially this may leave you feeling like you can't think straight, in the end these new neural circuits will actually leave your brain stronger.

It's a hormone thing

Many hormones are involved in maintaining a pregnancy and preparing the body for labor. Human chorionic gonadatropin is released as the embryo implants, causing a chain reaction that triggers production of estrogen and progesterone within the ovary; these, in turn, ensure that the uterus lining is not shed.

Growing a baby
involves every system
in your body.

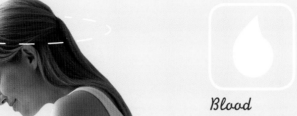

Blood

Your total blood volume rises
by 45 percent; most of this is
accounted for by extra fluid,
as your red blood cell mass
increases by just 20 percent.

Heart

Your stroke volume
(the amount of blood
pumped with each
heartbeat) increases
by 35 percent.

Hips and joints

The hormone relaxin
enables your pelvis to
widen so that it can
accommodate a baby.

Rib cage

Your ribs moves
out and upward, so
that you can inhale
more air. Your
diaphragm moves
upward, too.

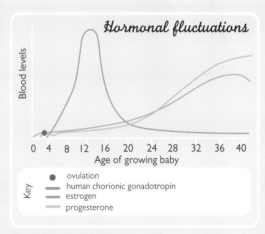

Hormonal fluctuations

Blood levels

0 4 8 12 16 20 24 28 32 36 40
Age of growing baby

Key
● ovulation
━ human chorionic gonadotropin
━ estrogen
━ progesterone

Belly-tastic

From about month
four your "thickened"
abdomen will start to
develop into a real
little belly bump!

Hormones

Your hormone levels will soar. During pregnancy,
you produce more estrogen in one day than you
ordinarily do in three years.

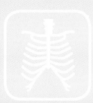

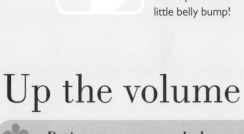

Up the volume

45%

During pregnancy your body sees a 45 percent rise in the volume of blood that flows through your veins.

First taste of *flavors*

Did you know that during pregnancy your baby can taste what you eat? Now, on today's in-utero menu…

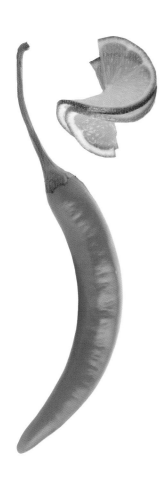

You may think your baby will have no concept of taste until he takes his first swallow of milk, or perhaps even when you start him on solid foods. But you may be surprised to learn that he will have experienced his first flavors as early as 13 weeks from conception, when his **taste buds** started to develop.

From 11 weeks your baby will learn how to swallow, and begin to gulp mouthfuls of the **amniotic fluid** that surrounds him in the uterus. The composition of amniotic fluid changes during the first trimester from a primarily water-based solution, similar to blood plasma, to one containing nutritional substances including carbohydrates, proteins, and fats, which contribute to his healthy growth and development. A baby will ingest significant quantities of this fluid each day, not only for hydration and nutrition, but also to practice the essential skills of swallowing and digesting. However, the amniotic fluid actually carries a **discernible flavor**, one that changes according to the foods eaten by the mother. So, once your baby's taste buds are sufficiently developed, he will be able to taste different flavors within the fluid, all influenced by the foods that you eat yourself.

The **taste receptors** that form on the baby's tongue develop quickly, as do the corresponding receptors in the nasal passages, providing a way for the baby to sense the fluid's taste and, crucially, its smell. It is believed that as much as 90 percent of a human's sense of taste is actually influenced by the smell receptors, and therefore it is the **strongly flavored foods**, such as spices, that are most readily conveyed to your baby.

Why not test this theory yourself? If you eat some spicy or pungent food and wait for about two hours, which is the time it takes for the flavor to reach the amniotic fluid, you might feel your baby respond, perhaps by hiccupping—you'll feel them as small, regular spasms—or even by wiggling around more than usual. On the other hand, your baby might be disappointingly unresponsive! Either way you don't need to worry, **strong flavors** won't distress your baby, they just help to provide him with more varied sensations to prepare for life on the outside.

In fact, researchers have noted that babies who are exposed to certain tastes in the uterus are **more eager to eat foods with that same flavor** once they have been born. A study conducted by researchers in Philadelphia examined a group of pregnant women by dividing them into three groups: one group drank a glass of carrot juice four times a week during pregnancy, and then switched to drinking just water once the babies had been born and were breast-feeding. The second group drank water during pregnancy and switched to carrot juice while they were breast-feeding. The last group avoided carrot juice entirely.

Strongly flavored foods with volatile compounds, such as those found in vegetables, fruits, garlic, and spices, transmit most easily into the amniotic fluid.

When the babies were weaned and just starting to eat solid foods, the researchers then offered them two kinds of cereal: plain and carrot-flavored. The babies who had been **exposed to carrot juice**, either via their mother's amniotic fluid or their breast milk, were more willing to eat the carrot-flavored cereal and were less likely to grimace than those babies who had never tasted carrot.

Further research has been done to test whether the smell transmitted to the amniotic fluid by certain foods was actually discernible. Researchers gave a group of pregnant women either garlic capsules or sugar capsules to swallow, and then took a sample of their amniotic fluid. When an independent group of people were asked to do a smell test, the samples from the women who had swallowed garlic capsules were readily detectable.

So, it seems you really are what you eat! And, strange as it may seem, whatever you put **on your menu** is not only filtering straight to your baby, but probably **influencing his future taste preferences** as well. French scientists did a study to support this idea: 12 pregnant women were given cookies and candy laced with aniseed during the 10 days or so leading up to birth. Hours after the women had given birth, their babies' reactions to the smell of aniseed were compared with babies who had not previously been exposed to the smell. Those who had sensed the strong flavor in the uterus seemed to like it more when presented with it after birth. The babies who had not been exposed to the flavor either reacted with disgust or indifference.

As an extension of this, prenatal and early postnatal exposure to a flavor is believed to enhance infants' enjoyment of that taste, both when starting solids and beyond into adulthood. This may go some way in explaining why different countries have specific cultural and ethnic preferences for cuisine and flavors. A Mexican child, for instance, will grow up with preferences for tastes that differ from those shown by a French, Chinese, or Indian child—and this predilection can, to an extent, be explained by their **exposure to those very first amniotic tastes**.

Maintaining a healthy and balanced diet during pregnancy is essential for nourishing your developing baby. However, by adhering to a varied diet you may well also be paving the way for your child to be born with an **innate enjoyment of healthy foods**. So next time you are rummaging in the fridge or cookie jar, spare a thought for the little one inside you. A potential sweet tooth could be substituted for a life-long love of broccoli if you play your cards right.

The risk roller coaster

You're delighted about your pregnancy, but suddenly so many everyday activities seem to pose a risk to you and your baby. But has life really become more hazardous?

Can I still take my allergy pills?

No, but talk to your doctor. Many antihistamines prescribed for allergy symptoms are safe during pregnancy, but your doctor may suggest a nasal spray or eye drops.

Can I still get a fake tan?

Yes, but skin can be supersensitive during pregnancy and may react to products even if you've used them before. Do a patch test and wait 24 hours before applying. The safest products are "paraben-free."

Can I still use the microwave?

Yes. There is no proof that microwave ovens pose a radiation risk or alter the nutritional value of foods.

Does smoking now and again really matter?

Yes. When you smoke (or inhale someone else's smoke), toxic chemicals including carbon monoxide pass into your bloodstream, reducing your baby's oxygen supply and harming the placenta. This can restrict your baby's growth and birthweight, make miscarriage more likely, and contribute to childhood asthma and infections. The good news? Quitting smoking benefits you and your baby instantly.

Is alcohol out of the question? Can I still have a

Do I have to stop eating Brie and Gorgonzola?

Can I take a flight during pregnancy?

Can I take a fake tan?

I had a few cocktails before I knew I was pregnant. Could I have harmed my baby?

Probably not. But don't waste time worrying about something you can't change. Alcohol crosses the placenta and enters the bloodstream of your developing baby, whose liver is too immature to break it down. So it's recommended you avoid alcohol entirely. Once you know that you're expecting, steer clear of alcohol and don't stress about the past.

Will I have to get rid of my cat?

No, but avoid dealing with cat litter (or wear gloves and wash your hands well) because of the risk of toxoplasmosis, a parasitic infection that can damage a baby's developing brain and eyes. A blood test can confirm whether you are immune already. Also avoid flea treatments (which contain insecticides). Instead, boil-wash your cat's bedding and treat your cat with regular shampoo.

What can I do about my cat? Are microwaves OK to use during pregnancy? Is the occasional cigarette so bad?

Is it safe to fly during pregnancy?

Yes, during your first two trimesters. After 36 weeks you may need a doctor's letter written within 72 hours to confirm your health and delivery date—check with the airline. If you're more than 28 weeks pregnant, it may be helpful to get a letter from your doctor confirming your due date and your fitness to fly.

Why can't I eat my favorite cheeses?

You may be able to, since pasteurized cheeses are perfectly safe. Pasteurized varieties of hard cheeses (like cheddar, Swiss and Parmesan) and soft cheeses (like Brie, Camembert and blue-veined cheeses) are sold in supermarkets and cheese stores nationwide. You're advised to avoid unpasteurized cheeses (check the label), These may contain *Listeria* bacteria, which in a tiny percentage of cases can lead to miscarriage or stillbirth.

Feeling *marvelous...*

Pregnancy triggers more hormonal action than any other life event. While some of the changes this promotes will be welcome—bouncy hair and even bouncier breasts—others can be less pleasing…

Fabulous hair

From the second trimester, people might start remarking on the thick, glossy appearance of your hair. This is due to raised levels of the hormone prolactin, which keeps your hair in a growth phase during pregnancy, meaning that it isn't shed as fast as usual.

What a glow

The pregnancy "glow" is no myth. When you're pregnant, your blood volume increases by 45 percent and your blood vessels also dilate, boosting the supply to your skin and securing that rosy complexion. Another happy consequence of this retained moisture is that it plumps out wrinkles, smoothing your skin.

Boob-tastic

Your breasts are likely to move up a cup size or two due to the ducts and tissue in your breast preparing for milk production. So enjoy your cleavage while you can!

Super stretchy

Can you bend deeper, twist further, and stretch more easily? The pregnancy hormone relaxin helps relax ligaments, while increased estrogen and progesterone soften connective tissue and loosen tendons. This increased mobility accommodates the growing baby and prepares your body for birth. Be wary of overstretching: increased ligament movement means less stable joints.

In the mood

Libido can fluctuate in pregnancy—at the beginning and end you may be too exhausted by the changes in your body to even contemplate sex, but your more "energetic" second trimester may be a golden opportunity. As an added bonus, the natural increase in blood flow and lubrication to your genitals, means that orgasms are easier to achieve and more intense. Happy days!

Nails may be extra glossy, long, and strong.

Breast tenderness felt early on should pass by the second trimester.

Nausea should fade after 12 weeks, leaving you to happily indulge in a varied pregnancy diet.

...or feeling *awful?*

Sufficient fluids and rest help combat swollen ankles and hands.

Gargling with salty water can keep softened gums healthy.

Stimulated oil glands can overproduce, causing acne.

 An entire human being is growing inside you, so it's no wonder at times you're floored with fatigue. Take this as a sign that your body needs rest and sleep.

What was I saying?

Impaired memory toward the end of pregnancy may correlate with a rise in sex hormones and their effect on the parts of the brain responsible for spatial memory.

All blocked up

An ongoing stuffy nose is experienced by up to 30 percent of pregnant women. This may be due to raised levels of estrogen and progesterone causing the mucous membranes and blood vessels of your nasal passages to swell, and produce more mucus.

Spitting blood

Increased blood flow and progesterone-triggered swollen or softened tissue can lead to sensitive, bleeding gums from the second trimester. Try a softer toothbrush, floss, and get dental checkups.

Skin pigmentation

In your second trimester, estrogen and progesterone cause an increase in levels of the pigment melanin. Moles and freckles may darken, as well as nipples and areolae. Many women also develop a dark strip (linea nigra) from the navel to the lower abdomen.

Cross those legs

With pregnancy comes an increased need to urinate. During your first trimester, you can blame the sharp rise in human chorionic gonadotropin, the hormone produced in response to the fertilized egg implanting in your uterus. An increased blood supply works the kidneys harder, too, making more urine. Later on, the urge to urinate returns as your expanding uterus puts pressure on your bladder.

Keep things moving

The relaxing effects of progesterone on your smooth muscle slows your digestion, which can result in constipation. Drinking lots of water and eating fiber-rich food can help things to keep moving.

My shoes don't fit!

Relaxin relaxes foot ligaments, which can elongate and flatten, and even move you up a shoe size (sometimes permanently). Shoes that support the arches help flat feet, as do those with wider laces or Velcro for fit-adjustment. Gel inserts are worth exploring.

Month 5

weeks 17–21

All about you

Clear to see
By now, your uterus is about the size of a melon and you probably have a visible bump. If this is a first pregnancy, this novel change in your shape is endlessly fascinating.

Getting higher
By the end of this month your uterus will reach—or grow above—your belly button.

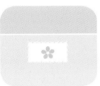

How stretchy?
Your skin is incredibly elastic thanks to the collagen and elastin fibers that make it flexible and firm; this elasticity means that it can stretch to accommodate your growing belly. It's quite common for skin on your belly to feel a bit itchy now and then, and you might want to start using a gentle emollient moisturizer daily.

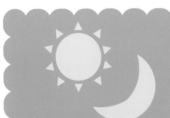

First routine
If you haven't already, you'll feel your baby move now as she takes up more space and the uterus walls stretch and thin. You may find she is lulled to sleep by your movements, and wakes when you rest.

Feet first
Relaxin production continues, which can actually cause your feet to grow a full size and make your joints even more flexible.

Sex on the menu

Some women have a renewed interest in sex now. High levels of estrogen and progesterone can bring a sense of well-being, while increased vaginal lubrication and blood flow to the pelvic area, as well as extra sensitivity in your breasts, can send your sex drive soaring. Some dads-to-be are nervous about having sex as their partner gets bigger and need reassuring that it's perfectly safe for the baby.

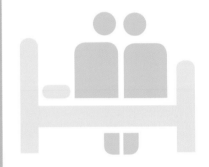

Your heart is working hard now. By the fifth month, cardiac output, or the quantity of blood your heart pumps a minute, has increased by 30 to 50 percent.

50%

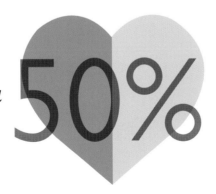

By this month
Your uterus will be about the size of a cantaloupe melon.

 At week 8

 At week 12

 At week 16

> **By about 18 weeks,** your baby actually outgrows the placenta, and continues to grow steadily.

Your growing baby

* Until nine or ten weeks, genitals are the same for girls and boys; but by 14 to 17 weeks, the reproductive structures will be complete and are often visible on an ultrasound scan.

* Myelin, a protective coating for your baby's nerves, a little like insulation on an electrical cord, is forming now. This encourages accurate transmission of nerve impulses.

* Your baby is laying down fat now, which will keep her warm, protect her muscles and bones, and provide her with the energy she needs to sustain her growth until she is born.

* By the end of this month, sweat and sebaceous oil glands are forming, and the top layer of her skin becomes more opaque.

* She is producing bowel movements (known as "meconium") now, but these are not released.

* Your baby inhales amniotic fluid as she practices breathing.

* She's very active in the uterus now, and her gymnastics will tone her muscles and make her stronger; if you haven't felt her before, you most certainly will now!

* At around 19 weeks, your baby will start to produce a white, waxy substance known as vernix, which covers the entire skin surface, protecting it and keeping it smooth and supple.

This month, think about...

* **Planning a vacation**
  If you're planning to fly later on, check the airline's policy and whether will you need a doctor's note after 36 weeks.

* **Checking out the unit**
  Tours at your local maternity unit allow you to check out facilities, such as labor rooms, and more mundane, but essential, details, such as parking facilities.

* **Getting up to speed**
  Have you considered a refresher childbirth course if this isn't your first pregnancy? Perhaps some advice has been updated, and it's often a good way to meet other new parents.

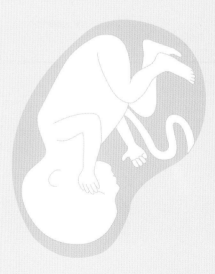

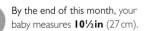

By the end of this month, your baby measures **10½in** (27 cm).

30   40   50

Your baby's first *home*

Designed to be the perfect place for your baby to grow, your uterus is an amazing organ. It performs an incredible range of functions from day one.

After conception, the **bundle of cells** that will become your baby journeys down the fallopian tube to the heart of your reproductive system: the uterus. This extraordinary organ's sole purpose is to ensure your baby's growth and delivery; encased within the pelvic cavity, it will **shelter and nourish** your baby for the following 40 weeks. Each month, the uterus anticipates a fertilized egg, and builds up its lining so the egg encounters a thick, spongy surface to nestle into. Once the fertilized egg has implanted, it triggers the release of high levels of progesterone, which maintains the uterine lining: your pregnancy is now underway.

Not only does the uterus provide an adaptable space for the tiny embryo to grow, it also builds a **complete life-support system**: shortly after the embryo beds down, designated cells start to form the placenta and umbilical cord, which link to your bloodstream, passing nutrients and oxygen to your baby and acting as his waste removal system. This organ with its thick muscular walls, supported by a hammock of ligaments, takes center stage now, and undergoes a series of dramatic changes to its size, shape, and position.

The hundreds of blood vessels supplying it enlarge, too, with some reaching 30 times their pre-pregnancy diameter, ensuring a **rich blood supply** to your baby.

With the onset of labor, triggered by the release of the hormone oxytocin, pressure in the uterus rises massively and its muscular walls contract with increasing intensity, exerting a huge force that eventually pushes your baby out into the world.

Did you know?

✳ On average, it takes six days for the fertilized egg to travel down the fallopian tube and implant in the wall of the uterus.

The uterine cavity expands from $^1/_{16}$ fl oz (4 ml) in its prepregnant state to 8 pints (4 liters) at term, encasing your baby in up to $3^1/_2$ pints (2 liters) of fluid.

✳ **Hormones thicken your cervical mucus, forming a plug at the entrance to your uterus to prevent any harmful bacteria from getting in.**

✳ A developing baby as young as 12 weeks old has been shown walking around the walls of his mother's uterus.

The fertilized egg is designed to attach to the walls of the uterus, since molecules on its surface stick to wall molecules. One scientist likened this to "a tennis ball rolling over a syrup-covered table."

✳ **After birth, the uterus returns to almost its pre-pregnancy size at a rapid rate: having taken 40 weeks to expand, it shrinks by half in just one week, and is virtually back to normal after six weeks—although it will always be a bit bigger than it started out.**

✳ Starting as an upside-down pear shape, the uterus resembles a watermelon by the end of pregnancy, having increased its weight from $2^1/_2$ oz (70 g) to an impressive 40 oz (1.1 kg).

Happy babymoon

Before embarking on the adventure of first-time parenthood, it is a good idea to take some time out for yourselves. Maybe this involves going on a last child-free vacation together, or just enjoying activities that will be more of a logistical challenge once your baby arrives.

If you intend to fly, schedule your trip for your second trimester, since this is the safest and most comfortable time to travel. A really long trip might be tiring and dehydrating so maybe spend more on accommodation than long-haul tickets, but if there is anywhere you are really eager to get to, then go for it. Avoid activities that could cause you to fall, such as skiing, cycling or horseback riding, for the remainder of your pregnancy. You need to strike a balance between staying fit and active, and ensuring rest and relaxation, since you need to conserve your energy for the new phase of life you are about to enter. Most importantly, spend time with your partner, talking and looking forward to the future, because you will inevitably have far less one-on-one time once you become new parents.

Stock up on sleep

Spend as much time as you can relaxing, daydreaming, and sleeping in. Find a shady hammock or lounge chair with a view and know that dozing is doing you lots of good.

Shop 'til you pop

Browse around stores while you only have yourself to please. Enjoy looking at gorgeous baby things, and plan which post-belly jeans to buy.

Catch up on culture

Dive into that book you've been meaning to read. Check out releases of new movies, visit art galleries, museums, and beautiful buildings.

Eat your heart out

Leisurely evening dinners will become more of a rarity once you're parents, so dress up, choose somewhere fantastic, and have a great meal.

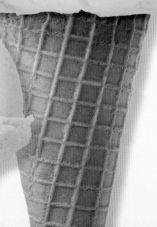

Natural wonders

Sit out under the stars, walk on the beach, and explore the countryside. Make the most of your flexibility before you need to find stroller-friendly paths and get your baby to bed at a sensible time.

Get pampered

Have a relaxing massage, facial, or maybe a pedicure so your feet look nice even if you can't see them. Many spas offer packages that are tailored for moms-to-be, as well as couples massage.

Up all night

Make the most of not needing a babysitter yet and stay up late, whether you see a band, musical, or play, or visit your favorite bar, restaurant, or nightclub.

Grown-up time

Spend time with your friends. Make sure they know how important they are to you, and then they'll be sure to understand if your catch-ups become less frequent while you find your parental feet.

Will I get
s-t-r-e-t-c-h m-a-r-k-s?

Nearly all pregnant women (up to 90 percent) will get stretch marks, but there is plenty you can do to reduce your chances and improve their appearance.

Whether you get stretch marks or not has more to do with **genetics** than expensive creams. If your mother had the kind of **elastic skin** that can accommodate a rapidly expanding body, maybe you have inherited it, too. These silver stripes of pregnancy—let's celebrate them as a **badge of honor**—appear when the body grows quickly and the skin tears a little as it races to catch up.

The stretch marks are actually scars in the skin's connective tissue, and while they never completely disappear, you can **reduce their development** and **improve their appearance**. It is important to drink plenty of water to **stay hydrated,** and eat healthily to nourish your skin. **Moisturizing your skin daily** will alleviate dryness along with any itchiness that you might be feeling, too. There is a huge range of moisturizers available for pregnant women, and you can choose from oils, body butters, lotions, and creams containing shea butter, olive oil, vitamin A and E, and other ingredients. Many are based on age-old remedies that are valued around the world (see opposite). If you do end up with stretch marks and want to remove them, the only **effective solutions** are topical application of tretinoin cream, laser treatment, or chemical peels. These options are OK only after pregnancy and breast-feeding, but don't rush to get treatment since most stretch marks fade over time. Most stretch-mark creams have an **uplifting or comforting scent** that helps to quell anxiety and enhance well-being, and the actual act of massaging is relaxing—and then perhaps the marks matter less anyway.

Natural remedies from around the world

✳ Cocoa butter, a fatty extract from the cocoa bean, was first used in Central America during the Mayan civilization as a skin healer, and is found in many moisturizing body butters. Cocoa also triggers the release of painkilling endorphins and the feel-good brain chemical serotonin.

Olive oil has been popular since ancient times in Greece and Italy as a means of preventing stretch marks, both when eaten and massaged into the skin. The constituent unsaturated fatty acid squaline, also found in human skin, boosts skin suppleness.

✳ Many women use creams for stretch marks that contain aloe (also called aloe vera) and it is also used for skin treatments in traditional Chinese medicine. Lotions made with aloe are safe for topical use during pregnancy. It's an ingredient that appears in many stretch-mark creams and lotions.

✳ Berber women use argan oil extracted from the seeds of a Moroccan tree. It is rich in antioxidants and omega-3 fatty acids. Rub it onto your skin.

Women in Polynesia and Micronesia use tamanu nut oil, thought to encourage the growth of new skin tissue.

Month 6

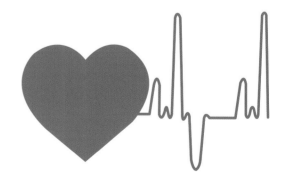

weeks 22–26

All about you

Rapid growth
You may be taken aback by the rate your belly is growing. By now, it's big enough to shift your center of gravity. Good posture and avoiding tilting your pelvis forward help keep you steady.

Taking care of your gums
The softening effect of progesterone that adapts your body so efficiently for pregnancy has some side effects, making your gums more susceptible to bleeding. Keep this in check with gentle, regular brushing.

Moving up
Your uterus is the size of a soccer ball now, and is rising steadily upward toward your ribcage.

Did I miss something?
Some experts believe that high levels of progesterone affect the way the brain works in pregnancy, causing forgetfulness. Others attribute any absentmindedness to the gaze turning inward, and women become increasingly preoccupied by what's going on in their body.

Pit stops
You'll grow accustomed to more frequent bathroom stops now as your uterus enlarges and presses on your bladder. Keep up the Kegel exercises to avoid leaks.

Just the two of us

Once you reach the third trimester, you may feel less inclined to venture out and happier to nestle in at home. Now—when you're not too big and feel surprisingly normal—is a good moment to enjoy some "couple" time, getting out on dates and away from daily distractions. If it's been a while since you both did something as normal as pop out for dinner, it can be refreshing to re-confirm your togetherness with a simple date.

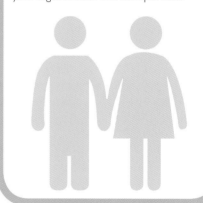

> Your blood pressure normally decreases during the second trimester. A typical reading is 105/70 mmHg.

At week 8   At week 12   At week 16

{ **Your baby** may already have a "favorite" hand, which is an early indication of left- or right-handedness. }

Your growing baby

* By 23 weeks, your baby is viable, which means she could survive outside of the uterus! The sucking reflex is developing, which will allow her to feed when she is born.

* Eyelashes, eyebrows, fingernails, and patterns of hair follicles on her scalp are all in place.

* Your baby's hearing is more sensitive and she may startle in response to loud noises. You may experience this as a sudden lurching feeling inside.

* Her eyes are now distinct, but they lack the pigment that will eventually give them color.

* She is flexing her muscles and experimenting with touch. She may grasp her umbilical cord or feel the surface of the uterus.

* She has a distinct sleep–wake cycle, moving and playing when she is awake. She'll drift quietly while she sleeps.

* The scrotum descends in boys.

By week 26
Your baby will be about the size of an iceberg lettuce.

This month, think about...

● *A good night's sleep*
While sleep is relatively settled now, experimenting how to get comfortable with one or two well-placed cushions and adopting relaxing practices, such as a warm bath 30 minutes before bed, puts in place strategies that will serve you well in the coming weeks.

● *Signing up child care*
This is the time to confirm child-care arrangements if you're returning to work fairly soon; or, if you're planning a longer break, start looking at the options.

● *Thought of a name?*
Fun though this undoubtedly is, it can take longer than you think and initiate some interesting debates—it might be worth starting the discussion now.

At week 21

By the end of this month, your baby measures **14 in** (36 cm) from crown to heel.

30   40   50

Baby's mini-*gymnastics*

Feeling your baby's tiny flutterings around 18–20 weeks is such a thrill. And in no time you'll feel that his movements become more definite, strong, and coordinated.

Your baby starts to make small movements, such as bending sideways, as early as seven to eight weeks. Over the next month or so, he progresses to being able to limber up his arms and legs as well as giving the occasional yawn. He will begin to flex and rotate his head—as if examining his internal world—and bring his hands up to touch his face, and have a really good stretch. That said, all such movements go unnoticed since he is too tiny and buried too deeply within the uterus's cushioning for you to be able to feel them.

Quick, quick, slow You might feel the first flutterings early on in your second trimester—like popcorn popping in your belly. The first flits and fidgets, known as "quickening," usually happen in the fifth month. Second-time moms often notice movements earlier partly as they know what to expect and partly because their uteruses are slightly thinner so movements are more easily felt.

Peak performance The perfect conditions for your would-be gymnast happen at 24–28 weeks, when he has plenty of amniotic fluid to move around in and is fairly high up in your uterus. For the next few weeks, you'll notice his moves become increasingly acrobatic—with somersaults, kicks, and punches built into the routine. You may start to wonder when your little karate kid is going to calm down, especially if he keeps you awake.

What was that? From about month seven, you may start to notice your baby startling at loud noises—it'll feel like a sudden jolt. You may recognize him hiccuping. Some babies hiccup and some never seem to at all; this variety is totally normal. Other jerky movements involve him swishing his head from side to side to find his thumb if it pops out of his mouth.

Ouch, that hurts! By the time you approach 36 weeks, his growing size and dwindling space will limit his movements, though you'll still feel him toss and turn. His growing muscles and developing brain mean he's become a mini Thai-style boxer: his kicks and punches become stronger and more coordinated. It's wonderfully comforting to feel a little prod from your baby but a kick under the ribs can be enough to make you jump in your seat. So, it's good to know that there's also less powerful bending and flexing of arms and legs going on, too.

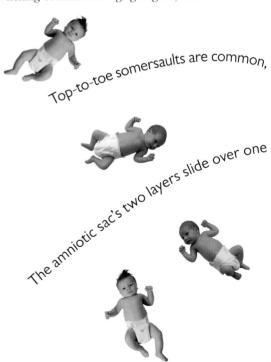

34 percent of all

Top-to-toe somersaults are common,

The amniotic sac's two layers slide over one

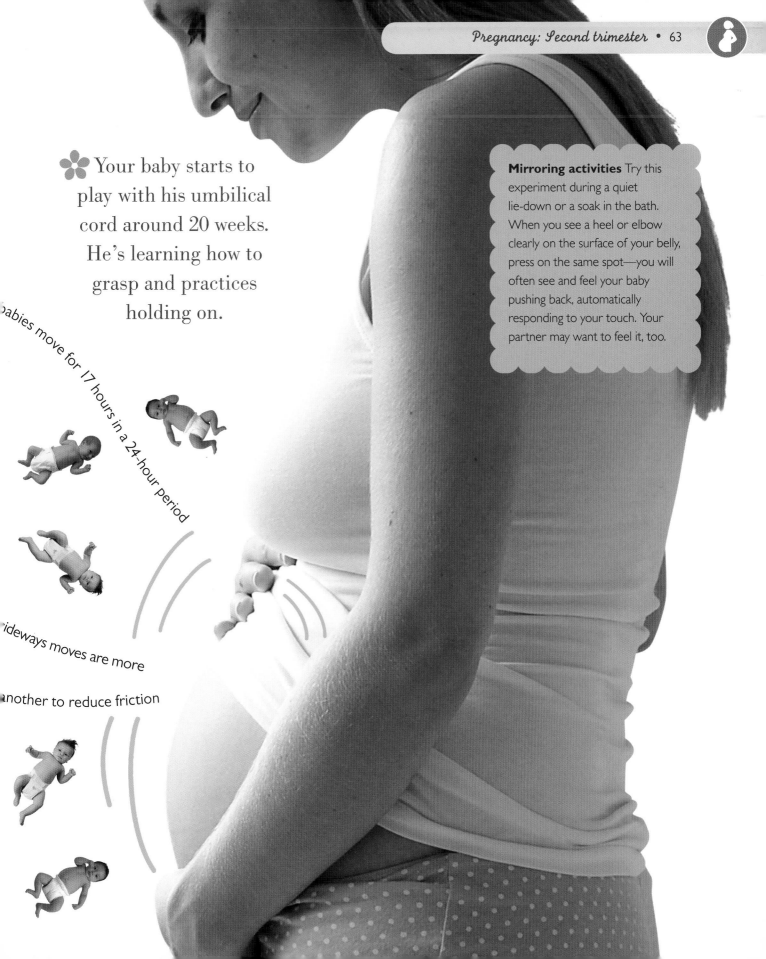

❀ Your baby starts to play with his umbilical cord around 20 weeks. He's learning how to grasp and practices holding on.

Babies move for 17 hours in a 24-hour period

Sideways moves are more

...another to reduce friction

Mirroring activities Try this experiment during a quiet lie-down or a soak in the bath. When you see a heel or elbow clearly on the surface of your belly, press on the same spot—you will often see and feel your baby pushing back, automatically responding to your touch. Your partner may want to feel it, too.

Your baby's *noisy* home

The drumbeat of your heart and the whoosh of your circulation make the uterus a noisy place to live, but your voice is your baby's favorite sound.

Your baby knows your voice over any other sound and will find it soothing, both in the uterus and once she is born. Research indicates that the mother's voice is the **dominant sound** in the uterus, so you can talk, sing, and whisper to your baby and she will most likely hear you. Your baby's ears will be structurally complete at about 24 weeks gestation, but tests have shown that some babies turn their heads in response to external sounds by 20 weeks. Your blood circulation, heartbeat, and breathing add up to an **ambient whooshing sound** that is louder to your baby than a nearby vacuum cleaner. Most of the external sounds she hears will seem low pitched, since being wrapped in the comfort of your uterus will **muffle any very loud sounds** and **harmful high frequencies**. Your baby will startle at loud noises such as a door slamming or a cough by moving around, registering a change in heart rate, or emptying her bladder.

She will have an appreciation for the subtleties of her **sonic environment**. Despite the fact that everything is muffled, it is likely that developing babies can tell the difference between people, and even between their **native language** and another one simply through the changes in **melody and rhythm**. A few weeks before birth, babies show a preference for their native language even when spoken by a stranger. And can you pave the way for a future musician during pregnancy? Music certainly **stimulates her developing brain**, but playing it through your pregnant belly may disrupt your baby's natural sleep patterns, and in turn her development. The general sounds from inside and outside your body are sufficient to stimulate your baby and she can enjoy your musical selection even if played across the room from her.

Did you know?

✳ Some parents report that their baby responds to loud rock music by kicking, and is calmed by soothing classical music. Music with a regular beat seems to be more calming than music with an irregular beat.

✳ Around 24 weeks, your baby can develop preferences for music that he will recognize after birth. Fetuses have even been observed moving to the beat in the uterus during scans.

{ *In Japan and China, it is believed that sound has a big influence on an unborn baby so disharmonious sounds are avoided. Some mothers tap gently on their pregnant belly to provide sound stimulation for baby.*

✳ For the first 16 weeks of your pregnancy, your baby will feel sound vibrations through his skin and skeletal tissues. He will be able to discern the patterns of voices as if they were music.

✳ The usual sound level in the uterus is around 75 decibels. To your baby this is the same volume you hear when driving with the car windows open. Imagine that whooshing sound!

✳ **Tests show that newborns prefer Mom's voice when passed through a filter that makes it sound as it would from the uterus.**

Pure indulgence

Whether you book yourself a professional session or treat yourself in the comfort of your own home, it's all about you, you, you.

Visit the professionals

Massage

If your muscles and joints are aching or you need an energizing boost, a hands-on therapy, such as professional pregnancy massage, can be just the tonic, as well as relieving stress and improving circulation. Some therapists use tables with a cutout for your belly so you can lie on your front for a full body massage, but you'll probably be most comfortable lying on your left side, supported by pillows; lying on your back or right side puts pressure on a major vein, which can make you feel light-headed.

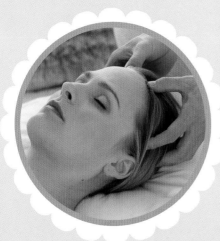

Indian head massage

If you prefer to sit during a professional therapy then why not consider an Indian head masage? It stems from Ayurvedic practice, which aims to balance the body, mind, and spirit. Expect a wonderful head, scalp, face, neck, upper arms, upper back, and shoulder massage. Research by the Institute of Indian Head Massage says massage can relieve headaches, congestion, and insomnia.

Reflexology

Designed to stimulate parts of the foot associated with different organs and glands, reflexology is best avoided in the first trimester with its higher risk of miscarriage, but some moms-to-be find it more relaxing than massage. A reflexologist will generally avoid stimulating the parts of the foot relating to the uterus and pituitary gland; except in the last week or so, when a session can bring on labor.

Don't go there!

✗ Deep tissue and sports massage is **too powerful** a type of massage when you're expecting, even on your legs.

✗ Steam rooms, saunas, and jacuzzis can **lower blood pressure and raise body temperature**, making you feel dizzy.

✗ In addition to raising body temperature, body wraps **contain chemicals** that can cross the placenta, so steer clear.

✗ Exposure to ultraviolet rays may be linked to the breakdown of folic acid so **don't use tanning beds**. Your skin is also more likely to burn when pregnant.

Beauty treatments

Waxing, facials, pedicures, and manicures are all safe during pregnancy, though your skin might feel more sensitive than usual, so mention your pregnancy (if it's not obvious) to your therapist.

1
Create the atmosphere
Put on some music, get out some fresh towels, and dim the lights to create a calm, relaxing environment in your bathroom or bedroom.

2
Take a soak
Run a bath and surround the tub with a few candles, if you choose. Scented candles are OK, if you prefer an aroma, but don't add essential oils to the bathwater; they should be avoided during pregnancy, because not enough research has been done to verify their safety.

3
Moisturize from head to toe
Use a rich, natural body cream all over, especially on your elbows, feet, and hands.

4
Pamper your hands and feet
Give yourself a manicure and pedicure. Remove nail polish and wash your hands with gentle, organic soap and soak them in warm water. Buff your nails to a shine. If you are having a scheduled cesarean, don't apply nail polish since doctors observe your nails for paleness during surgery.

5
Give yourself a facial
Exfoliate and cleanse your skin for a mini facial. Your skin may be feeling extra sensitive or dry at the moment and you may want to switch to natural products during your pregnancy. Pregnancy hormones can cause acne and darker patches (chloasma) and gentle facials might help alleviate these. Facial oils can rehydrate and balance sensitive skin.

6
Cocoon and relax
Wrap yourself in a robe or large towel and relax with a magazine or take a nap.

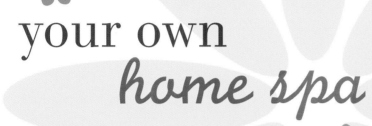

your own
home spa

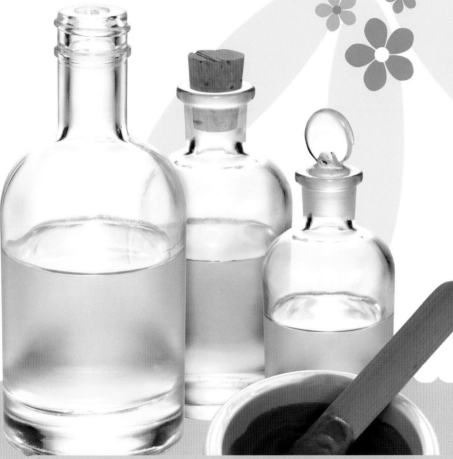

Homemade mask

Face masks are easily whipped up in the kitchen. Why not try one based on yogurt, which cools and moisturizes?

Just give me *a list!*

You may find your jaw dropping when you write out lists of what you need to amass for your tiny unborn child. It's a good idea to decide in advance what you need to get you through the first few weeks.

STARTER GEAR— **ESSENTIALS**

HAVE THE FOLLOWING READY FROM THE BEGINNING:

 Newborn-size diapers and a changing mat.

 Baby wipes, balls or pads of cotton, or cloths.

 6–8 sleepsuits and the same of onesies, a cardigan or coat, and a summer or winter hat.

 8–10 cotton burp cloths.

 Bottles, nipples, formula, and cleaning equipment if you're bottle-feeding.

 Moses basket or crib; cotton sheets and swaddles and/or sleep sacks.

 Newborn car seat.

 Baby stroller.

20,000

A clean bottom!
Wipes, cotton balls, or cloths are your diaper changing arsenal. While wipes are convenient, over diaper-changing years you could use a staggering 20,000!

DID YOU KNOW?
Wipes are often claimed to dry out delicate newborn skin, yet a recent UK study found that one sensitive-skin brand was as hydrating as cotton balls and water.

In the US, over 7.5 billion lbs of disposable diapers are thrown away every year.

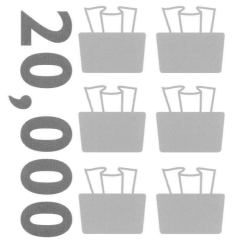

4–10 PER DAY ✕ **2.5 YEARS** = **6,000**

Diapers, diapers everywhere
Whether disposable or reusable, these are part of life now. For a few months, your baby will use 10 diapers a day, and 4–6 a day after that. Until you toilet train at around two and a half years, you'll use around 6,000 disposable diapers.

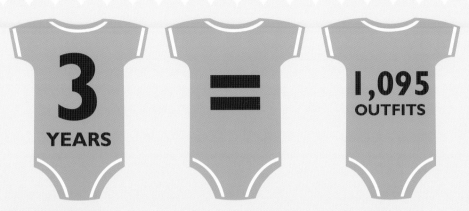

3 YEARS = **1,095 OUTFITS**

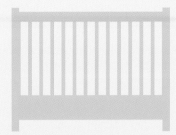

First wardrobe

Your newborn's needs are simple: sleepsuits and onesies will be pretty much all she wears at first. Second-hand baby clothes are a godsend: cheap (or free) and usually in nearly perfect condition. She'll get through at least one outfit a day, amounting to 1,095 outfit changes over three years!

Sound asleep

Moses baskets are cosy, light to carry, and ideal in the early weeks when a crib can seem enormous compared to your baby. You'll need two to three fitted sheets, plus swaddles or sleep sacks to keep your baby warm. However, Moses baskets are quickly outgrown, and then you'll need to upgrade to a crib, which should accommodate your baby for the first two years. As long as it conforms to safety standards, it can be second-hand, but buy a new mattress because a second-hand one can harbor dust and dampness, and may lack sufficient support for your baby's back.

Getting around

Your infant car seat will snap into a stroller or special frame, which makes it easy to remove a sleeping baby from your car and push him to your next destination without waking him. When your baby can sit upright, switch to an umbrella-style stroller or use the matching stroller that came with your travel system.

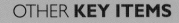

OTHER KEY ITEMS

 Baby monitor
Being able to hear what is going on in baby's room can be a great comfort.

 Bouncy chair
Ideal for gently rocking and containing a small baby.

 Baby bath
These are useful, but a sink does the job just as well in the early weeks.

 Changing bag
A compartmentalized bag can do wonders for your organization.

GLOBAL TRENDS

Many parents invest in a sling. Super convenient, these leave hands free and baby comforted. Also, many dads enjoy the bonding opportunity they provide.

Now popular in the West, slings have been used for centuries in developing countries.

In the car

If you drive (or even if you are planning on leaving the hospital in a taxi), you will need a newborn rear-facing car seat. A second-hand seat isn't recommended, unless you know its history and are confident it hasn't been in an accident. Between one and two years old, your baby will move into a forward-facing seat.

The third trimester
In the *home stretch*

In the last three months of pregnancy your baby is getting fatter, longer, and bigger all around, and you'll clearly see your belly expanding and feel it becoming heavier now. It's natural to feel an urge to slow down and get things together for the countdown to birth and new motherhood. Enjoy this time to prepare for your baby's arrival, both mentally and practically—if you haven't started equipping your home then now's the time. As your body accommodates your ever-growing baby, you might find that you start to walk differently as your center of gravity shifts— who's ready for the pregnancy waddle?

Congratulations! You are almost there.

Only about 5 percent of babies are born on their due date.

WOMEN gain an average of 11 lb (5 kg) in the third trimester.

Your baby's eyes open at around 28 weeks.

THE HORMONE RELAXIN causes your feet to become longer and wider, a change that may become permanent.

Your baby drinks and then urinates in the amniotic fluid; the whole volume of amniotic fluid recirculates every two to three hours.

You're likely to recall dreams vividly because pregnancy symptoms wake you frequently from sleep.

Your baby is piling on the fat and in the final ten weeks gains half of his final full-term weight.

IN ANCIENT ROME, WOMEN WERE GIVEN A DRINK made from powdered sows' dung to relieve pain in labor. Feel like adding that to your birth plan?

At 32 weeks, your baby can suck, which means that if born now, he would be able to feed.

Some 80 percent of dads-to-be fear that they won't be able to be useful enough when their partner is in labor.

Your baby's intestines are lined with a thick, greenish black, sticky substance known as meconium, which will become his first and stickiest stool.

IN CHINA, ACUPUNCTURE IS USED INSTEAD OF EPIDURAL ANESTHESIA in 98 percent of vaginal births.

At 40 weeks, the placenta is the size of a large dinner plate.

A NEWBORN BABY is able to stick out his tongue to mimic someone else sticking out their tongue.

Month 7

All about you

Working overtime
Your circulation and other body systems are working at a fantastic rate to meet the increasing demands of your expanding uterus and growing baby. Regular naps now are almost medicinal in their ability to re-energize you.

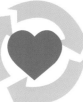

Thinking ahead
The amazing placenta protects your baby beyond pregnancy as it starts to pass on antibodies to prepare her for life in her new world.

Your changing breasts
Your nipples and areolae (the area around them) may become larger and darker, which some experts believe makes it easier for your baby to locate when she is born.

A little at a time
Weight gain actually slows down a little now, but because your uterus presses on your stomach, you fill up more easily, so eating little and often is easier than having a main meal.

A bit of a squeeze
Your uterus is about 4–4½in (10–12cm) above your navel now, and weighs about 2lb (1kg). While its expansion accommodates your baby, it presses on your diaphragm, which can make you feel a bit breathless.

Getting organized

You've done the spreadsheet, now it's time to put systems in place so that you don't have to worry about paperwork when concentrating on your new baby. Marvel at your efficiency by setting up direct debits for regular payments, compiling internet supermarket lists so that you can restock at the push of a button, and creating a reminder system so that dry cleaning gets picked up, library books returned, and the bills get paid on time.

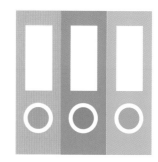

By the end of the seventh month you have gained around 15 lb (7 kg); total weight gain by the end of pregnancy is around 29 lb (13 kg).

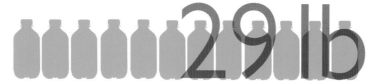
29 lb

By week 30
Your uterus will be about the size of a medium pumpkin.

 At week 8

At week 12

 At week 16

0 (cm)   10   20

Your growing baby

✳ The buds of your baby's baby teeth have been in place since week six of pregnancy; her permanent teeth are starting to form now.

✳ Between 26 and 30 weeks, your baby's eyes, which have been fused firmly shut to protect them and help them develop, begin to open. She can see! By 27 weeks, they have a little pigment, too.

✳ Lanugo (downy hair on baby's body) starts to disappear yet this can take most of the third trimester, so she may be born with patches.

✳ She kicks vigorously now, and her arms and legs will begin to pull up toward her chest to allow her to adopt a comfortable position for the duration of your pregnancy.

✳ Her lungs are producing a substance called surfactant, which lubricates the smallest parts of the airways (alveoli). If born now, she would stand a good chance of being able to breathe on her own.

✳ The brain grows more now, and starts to fold over to fit in the skull, forming its characteristic grooves and wrinkles.

✳ The average baby weighs 2⅞lb (1.3 kg) by the end of month seven.

✳ Your baby's bone marrow now takes over the job of creating red blood cells that transport oxygen around her body.

✳ Wrinkles disappear as skin begins to smooth out as fat is laid down.

This month, think about...

● **Time for essentials**
Onesies, sleepsuits, bottles, diapers, bedding, and cleaning equipment will be needed—start stockpiling now!

● **Want a water birth?**
If you'd like a water birth, but haven't looked into one, it's not too late. Your doctor might refer to you a specific hospital or birthing center in your area.

● **Wrapping up work**
Is everything in place at work to hand over? Have you talked to your employer about your plans for returning?

● **Budgeting ahead**
Thinking about your weekly budget now and the reality of a belt-tightening period may help you see where to make savings.

As you enter your third trimester, your baby takes center stage: her rapid growth and preparation for birth mean you need to take it easier now.

 At week 21

 At week 26

By the end of this month, your baby measures **15¾in** (40 cm) crown to heel.

30   40   50

What do *babies do* all day?

In addition to the all-important matter of sleep, your baby's days are full of variety—from dreaming and exploring his environment to practicing stretching and listening to the sounds of his world.

 ### Big yawn

Your baby started to yawn at just 11 weeks of development, and he does it about twice as much as an adult. Just like us, yawns are accompanied by stretching, and they tend to happen when he is entering a more active period—in essence, he is test-driving the process of waking up.

 ### Practice makes perfect

As your baby cycles through the different sleep states and waking periods, he is stimulating all the various parts of his brain and giving his nervous system a workout, ready to tackle the upcoming challenges of life.

 ### Wakey wakey

During his waking hours, your baby will explore his environment through touch, flexing and extending his body, bringing his hands and feet together, and even grasping his umbilical cord. Luckily later-born children will apparently have more room to tumble and turn since the uterus has been previously stretched.

 ### Getting ready to go out

As birth gets closer, your baby will cut down his nap times to a mere 85 percent of his time, just like a newborn. By 32 weeks, his brain and nervous system will be as developed as it will be at birth.

 ### Mommy and me

Your baby is being bathed in your hormones, so your habits and emotions influence his rhythms. High levels of stress hormones will increase his activity. In contrast, it seems that your baby will automatically relax (his heart rate will slow) when he hears your voice.

 ### Dream on, dreamer

By the beginning of the final trimester your baby will be having organized patterns of sleeping and waking, including periods of REM sleep, indicating that he is dreaming. What he dreams about is a mystery, but he is probably rehearsing movements he's learned or reliving the sensations of life in the uterus.

 ### Out of sync

You may think that your baby starts kicking just when you want to get some sleep, but the more likely explanation is that he is stretching now that you have reclined and are comfy, and your abdominal muscles have relaxed, giving him a bit more room to maneuver.

 ### Right on schedule

Once you and your baby have met, you can start to lay the foundations of a future routine. Exposing him to lots of light during the day and keeping it dark at night should start to give his body the general idea.

While you may be struggling to get comfortable enough to sleep, your baby will be having no such trouble—spending on average 90–95 percent of his time dozing.

90–95%

Intestines

From the second trimester, the intestines are up and running, making meconium—a green–black sludgy mixture of hair, dead skin cells, bile, and amniotic fluid.

Kidneys

From about week 21, your baby is swallowing amniotic fluid. His kidneys filter this and produce urine, albeit weak, which is then urinated into the amniotic fluid. And the process starts again.

Legs

In addition to karate kicks and the more balletic bends and flexes, your baby will also enjoy walking around the inside of your uterus.

Lungs

From about week 17, your baby is practicing breathing, but with amniotic fluid instead of air. About week 28, his lungs start to produce surfactant, which inflates the lungs after birth.

Hands and arms

While awake, your baby is busy feeling his face and body, grasping the cord, and sucking a thumb.

Eyes

Once his eyelids open, at about 27 weeks, your baby will start to open his eyes when active and close them during sleep.

Brain

The number of connections in his brain is increasing all the time. And he's developing basic reflexes and patterns of activity and resting.

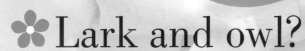

❁ Lark and owl?

Your baby's schedule doesn't reflect the cycle of the day and night until at least a month or two after birth.

Facts about *diapers*

There is a vast array of diapers available today—you can choose between disposables, cloth or reusables, biodegradables… or you may even attempt to avoid diapers altogether.

What are the options?

Disposable

The most absorbent type of diaper, disposables are convenient, portable, widely available to buy, and don't contribute to your laundry. They contain ultra-absorbent polyacrylates—when they get wet these chemicals turn into gel, holding the wetness away from your baby's skin and minimizing the risk of diaper rash. However, disposable diapers are not good for the environment—they take 200 years or more to decompose in a landfill, and one baby can generate hundreds of dirty diapers in a year. They are also expensive to buy.

Reusables

Reusable cloth diapers work out to be cheaper than disposables. You pay more initially but the costs are lower overall, and are even a better value if you have more than one child. Modern designs are easy to change and wash, but they are less absorbent than disposables so need to be changed more often. Some washable diapers have a removable liner, so you don't have to wash the whole diaper each time. While you use large amounts of energy washing and possibly drying, you will save hundreds of diapers from going into a landfill.

Biodegradable

Eco-friendly diapers are easy to use, chemical- and bleach-free, and use cotton padding to absorb liquid instead of polyacrylates. They are slightly more expensive than non-eco diapers, and while they can be composted they still take around 50 years to break down in a landfill.

No diaper approach

Some parents try and learn to read their baby's signs that he needs to "go," and then quickly usher him to a toilet in time. Gradually he learns to control this himself, often earlier than children who are used to wearing diapers (see also pages 278–279).

OTHER EQUIPMENT

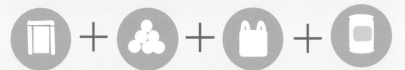

CHANGING MAT
A padded, wipeable changing mat offers a hygienic, comfortable space to change your baby's diaper.

WIPES
Use wipes or moist, soft washcloth to clean the diaper area.
.

CHANGING BAG
A bag that can be streamlined for when you are out and about can help you keep organized.

DIAPER CREAM
If your baby's bottom is red or sore, a thin layer of diaper cream will heal and protect the area.

Diaper facts

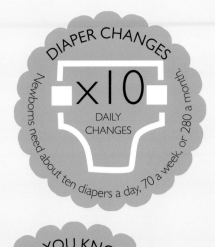

DIAPER CHANGES
×10
DAILY CHANGES
Newborns need about ten diapers a day, 70 a week, or 280 a month.

DID YOU KNOW?
In 2008, disposable diapers comprised 2.3 percent of landfill waste in the US.
3 billion
DIAPERS ARE THROWN OUT IN THE UK EVERY YEAR.

GLOBAL TRENDS
The global market for disposable diapers is rapidly expanding—it is due to reach a turnover of $33.4 billion per year by 2017.
In 2012, the no-diaper approach is popular with celebrities.

You may prefer to have a flexible approach and use a combination of diaper types.

REALITY **CHECK**

 Environmental impact

The debate about which diaper is most eco-friendly is ongoing, and the fact is whichever kind of diaper you use, you will have an impact on the environment. You can reduce your carbon footprint by using a lower temperature to wash reusables, and line drying rather than using a tumble dryer. Choose biodegradable diaper liners for reusables. If you use disposables, only change when necessary and look for good deals on more eco-friendly brands.

Save and strengthen *your back*

As you move into the third trimester your back needs all the support it can get. So, it's time to make your back an everyday priority and start showing it some tender loving care.

During the third trimester, the volume and weight of your expanding belly causes a shift in your center of gravity. To counteract this, you may notice the curve of your back becomes accentuated and you'll naturally lean backward. While this helps your stability, leaning causes back and shoulder muscles to work harder and can result in pain.

Everyday back care

Think about your back as you go about your day. Be careful as you lift a child to prevent straining your back. If you have to carry heavy bags, carry the weight evenly between both arms.

Wear supportive, low-heeled shoes that distribute your weight equally.

Maintain your good posture to let your muscles support you as well as they can; stand up straight and tall, and keep your shoulders back and relaxed.

Bend your knees and keep your back straight when you're picking something up but, of course, ask someone else to lift anything heavy.

Sit on a birthing ball instead of the sofa to watch TV. It offers back-building benefits while you catch up on the latest news or miniseries. Your body has to work to keep stable on the ball, and this helps to improve your core strength.

Support your back while you sleep by keeping your knees bent, and use pillows under and around your belly or knees to feel comfortable. If your mattress feels too soft, firm it up with a board underneath.

Staying active

Gentle exercise can help to both alleviate lower back pain and to improve the strength in your back. A study in the *International Journal of Gynaecology and Obstetrics* showed that women who exercised three times a week for 12 weeks during the second half of pregnancy had less severe lower back pain.

Swimming is the ideal exercise for late pregnancy because it supports your body weight, takes pressure off your back, and improves muscle tone and strength. It's wise to avoid breaststroke, though, if you have any pelvic pain.

Relaxin's effect on your ligaments is in full flow, readying your pelvis for birth. Your back is less stable and abdominal muscles find it harder to support your back, too.

Paying attention to your posture will reap rewards when it comes to preventing back pain.

Shoulders
Your back muscles work hard to pull on your shoulders to help keep stable. Remember to keep them relaxed and not hunched up.

Back
Don't be tempted to exaggerate your curve further, your body's already doing what it needs to.

Hips
Keep your hips square and tuck your bottom under when standing.

Knees
When standing, keep your knees soft and apart. Avoid crossing your knees when sitting down, too.

Feet
Stand with your feet hip-width apart and flat on the floor. The same goes for sitting.

Working back muscles
Since your back muscles are working so hard to keep you upright and stable, they'll need a good stretch most days.

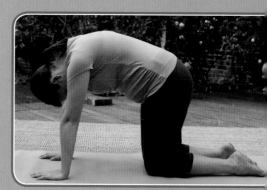

Cat stretch
To ease away aches and pains, this back stretch also reinforces a connection with your abdominal muscles.

1) Start on all fours with your knees directly under your hips and hands under your shoulders. Point your fingers forward and keep your neck in line with your body.

2) Breathe in as you pull in your abdomen and round your back upward as far as you feel is comfortable, and allow your neck and head to relax gently forward. Don't lock your elbows. Hold for five seconds.

3) Breathe out as you relax your abdomen and back, slowly returning to a flat back. Repeat slowly up to ten times.

Pelvic tilt
You can do this sitting back stretch any time anywhere, so no excuses.

1) Sit up straight on a chair with your feet shoulder-width apart on the floor.

2) Tighten your belly button in toward your spine, and press your back into the back of the chair. Hold for five seconds, then relax a little. Repeat up to ten times.

Best-laid *plans*

Now may be the time to set aside any urge to control events
and embrace the uncertainties of birth and parenthood.

As a pregnant woman you will be encouraged to write a birth plan as a way of mentally preparing for childbirth and the many decisions it involves: what do you need to do to feel confident and safe? How will you cope with pain? Who will support you through labor? Your ideal plan might involve a water birth at home with only scented candles and relaxing music for pain relief. So, how will you cope if you never even get to fill the pool, but are rushed to hospital for an emergency cesarean? When **expectations are not met**, feelings of helplessness, frustration, humiliation, even incompetence and guilt can follow. And a loss of self-esteem can be damaging at this vital cusp of new life.

It's good to make plans. A birth plan prompts you to weigh the pros and cons, educate yourself about options, and make informed choices—in short, it encourages you to take an **active part in the birth process**. The birth plan was first championed by pioneering childbirth educator Sheila Kitzinger in the 1970s as an **empowering tool** designed to give parents input into their obstetric experience. Studies show that they make women more aware of their options, provide the language to communicate effectively with staff, enhance confidence in labor, and lead to a more satisfying experience, which, in turn, supports positive interactions in the early weeks of life.

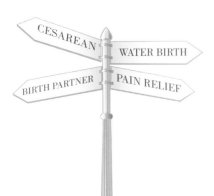

But planning an ideal birth does not necessarily mean you will get one. Studies have looked at the forces that shape **women's choices in pregnancy**: they've changed since the 1970s. Now there is widespread acceptance of cosmetic surgery and loss of belief in the "art of suffering"; this may encourage expectations for a pain-free makeover-style scheduled "life event," rather than an unscheduled biological process. Celebrity culture contributes to the notion that there's a good way to give birth (and shrink to size four in weeks), while supermarket shopping sets up the assumption that everything

> Some studies show that women who remember their birth experience in a positive light are more likely to have a subsequent child more quickly.

in life should be easier, quicker, and more convenient. Then there's our human respect for the consumer's right to have what we want when we want. If such assumptions underpin our wishes and hopes for one of the most important days of our lives, it's no wonder a birth plan can set us up to fail.

Birth plans can't lead to specific birth outcomes. What they can do is **encourage you to be realistic** about pregnancy and your birth choices, and, crucially, give you the confidence to make new decisions if your circumstances suddenly change. Studies show that couples who go into childbirth having attended birth-preparation classes and having made a birth plan feel more prepared and are more likely to perceive the experience as positive (albeit painful). And how a mother experiences and remembers the birth has a huge effect on her **self-confidence as a parent**.

Human beings have a need to tell stories about important life events, since it helps us understand our changing roles and relationships. Birth not only brings a child into the world, it also **creates new parents**, and the stories we tell each other about the birth help define the parents we become. But what if your birth story doesn't follow the much hoped-for, positive formula? What if your experience was bad, or even traumatic? Everyone loves the thrill of a horror story, but if that's what you remember and recount about the birth of your child, it's useful to refocus the narrative so that you don't end up retelling a negative story.

Constantly repeating a traumatic tale can leave a negative emotional imprint that studies suggest can have serious consequences for family relationships.

Just as planning the perfect birth can lead to a fall, **planning to be a perfect mother**—or even believing that she exists—can do the same. That woman who blooms through pregnancy, has a tear-free birth, a baby who feeds well and sleeps through the night from six weeks, and total confidence in her parenting ability is, thankfully, just a myth—but she will undermine you if you let her.

There are many **different styles of parenting** (see pages 168–169) and different ones suit different people. But even once you have established the style that suits you, it won't always be the best way to handle your child— sometimes it will work, sometimes you will have to rethink your approach. The road is never smooth.

That's tough news when so many of us wait until later in life to have kids, once we have a good job, a great partner, a lovely home, and are used to getting what we want. Pregnancy and parenting don't follow those rules. The least

> Labor and birth can be unpredictable, so a birth plan should be flexible.

stressful approach is to let go of assumptions, **expect everything to change** all the time, and be open to rethinking your best-laid plans. You'll have an easier ride if you accept that an ideal is impossible, it's OK not to be the perfect parent, and fine if things don't go as planned. Honing your ability to welcome the unexpected gives an opportunity to gain in experience. Positivity, mingled with realism, helps, as does having an enormous amount of compassion for yourself, your partner, and your beautiful child.

GREAT BIRTH

Busy doing nothing

Hopefully you are reading this lying on the sofa, feeling calm and rested; but if you are finding the last months of pregnancy anything but relaxing, you'd better think about setting aside some "me time."

Escaping from the stresses and strains of everyday life—even for just 15 minutes—not only has body-wide benefits for you but also calms your baby and boosts her well-being.

In bed or feet up on the sofa? No matter where you choose to unwind, it's a great habit to block out 15 or 20 minutes each day for relaxing. The best time of day to sit or lie down and relax is when you feel a natural dip in your energy levels—it might be after lunch or in the early evening.

In your mind's eye Visualization exercises can de-stress you; just feel the tension slipping away. Some take practice while others are quick to follow. Try this short one. Lie on your bed or sofa, close your eyes, and imagine a door in front of you. Go through it, leaving all worries behind you, and find a quiet place such as a beautiful garden, tropical beach, or fragrant meadow. After a few minutes, go back through the door. Wiggle your fingers and toes to come around and energize yourself again.

And now relax… Classes that teach you how to relax can be beneficial in pregnancy and for the forthcoming labor, too. Pregnancy yoga teaches breathing awareness and how this can relax your body. Hypnobirthing teaches simple but specific self-hypnosis, relaxation, and breathing techniques for a relaxed birth. You're not in a trance, but are aware, calm, and able to talk.

Return to the uterus For a glimpse into your baby's world, arrange a flotation session where you float effortlessly in the quiet and dark, in body-temperature warm water, and unwind physically and mentally. It's safe during pregnancy and can relieve a backache as well as neck and shoulder tension.

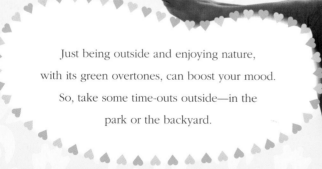

Just being outside and enjoying nature, with its green overtones, can boost your mood. So, take some time-outs outside—in the park or the backyard.

Learning how to relax during your pregnancy will be an invaluable skill to call upon during labor.

Relaxing is not just about lying down; regular exercise during pregnancy helps relieve aches and pains and triggers the release of mood-enhancing endorphins.

Acupuncture

Using tiny specialized needles inserted at specific points to realign energy pathways in the body, acupuncture can re-energize you if fatigue is problematic, lessen any nagging back pain, and even turn a breech baby.

Switch to juices A juicer is a great investment during pregnancy, since you can give yourself a boost of vital vitamins and energy from a range of fruits and vegetables. Tangy flavors can help keep pregnancy sickness at bay, and juices won't leave you edgy and wired like caffeine-based beverages.

Plug into your mp3 Put together a playlist of relaxing music that you can listen to for 20 minutes or so each day. Soothing music can release endorphins, calm the mind, and distract you from work or other concerns; and if you play it out loud your baby gets to appreciate your musical selection too. Music can be a powerful trigger to calm and relax you and can be a useful tool—or distraction—during labor and birth.

On vacation "Babymoons" started out as vacations you take with your partner and new baby. But the idea has become popular as a vacation you take before your baby arrives (see page 56) as a special time to promote bonding and togetherness with your partner.

Expert attention Many therapies offer great benefits during pregnancy, and having an hour or so to yourself with healing hands can be priceless. Choose from a host of therapies—but always see a professional therapist and always tell them you are pregnant. A professional pregnancy massage can melt away muscle aches as well as promote sleep and relaxation. Osteopathy also uses massage but with manipulation, and gentle stretching, to help your body work more efficiently and relieve pubic and back pain. The Alexander Technique focuses on posture, and regular sessions can counter backaches and fatigue.

Information *overload?*

It seems as if everybody thinks they know how to raise your child. There is so much information to sift through, how do you choose what to believe?

By now you probably feel **bombarded with information** from baby-care websites, blogs, books, family, friends, and even strangers who feel compelled to offer you unsolicited advice at the supermarket. There will be recommendations, advice, and warnings on where and how to give birth, what you need to buy, and how best to nurse, bathe, clothe, and change your new baby. To confuse things further, much of this information is contradictory, and you can end up feeling like an incompetent parent before you've even started. So, how to best sift through and make sense of everything? And who are these experts undermining our confidence and mystifying child care? **Government advice** on parenting changes over time and from country to country, often to reflect political pressures. **Child-care experts** often disagree with each other over the basics, from sleep strategies to discipline. **Research scientists** have agendas, as do the media, and **friend and family opinions** are just that.

In short, there is often no "right way." The best parents have confidence, warmth, and a relaxed attitude that comes from experience. So, how can you develop that confidence? There's no alternative to spending huge amounts of time—day and night—getting to know your baby. And while it's good to take advice from people whose values you trust, remember that when it comes to your body and your baby, **you are the best judge**. Inevitably there will be times when things don't go quite as planned, but by learning from mistakes, you'll figure out what best suits you and your new family. Be confident in your **parental instinct**—it is fully primed ready for action, even before your baby is born.

Taking advice from the experts

* In a 2002 study, 71 percent of parents questioned said they got their parenting information from books, TV, magazines, and videos; only 50 percent consulted their mother or mother-in law.

Parenting experts go in and out of fashion. Dr. Benjamin Spock was the first best-selling parenting author, and he led the way for books authored by doctors, nannies, psychologists, and celebrities. Your parents probably followed different "experts" than you will.

* Read a few parenting books and websites until you find approaches that suit you. And feel free to pick and mix from many different practices.

* Ask your doctor where she gets her advice—guidelines for health professionals tend to bring together the results of clinical trials and real clinical experience with individuals and communities. But there won't be guidelines for all parenting issues, such as sleeping or child care.

If you know what you value and are clear about the rules you want to live by, you'll feel better equipped to evaluate others' advice. Don't assume your partner has the same ideas, so make time to discuss as much as possible.

* Researchers have been looking into whether parents are the deciding factor in a child's future success and happiness; some studies show that a child's peers may have just as great an influence.

Month 8

weeks 31–35

All about you

Almost there...

You're in the home stretch... and may start to feel a little jittery—elated one minute, anxious the next. Your emotions are affected, too, by hormone levels starting to peak as labor approaches.

Extra fluids

Blood volume rises into late pregnancy, helping your body support your baby on this final stretch. A possible secondary effect is that fluid seeps into tissues, causing swelling. Putting your feet up helps to reduce swelling, and—although it sounds counterintuitive—drinking lots of water helps your kidneys flush out excess fluid.

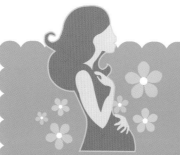

Preparing for labor

As your uterus prepares for its big moment, you may notice stronger Braxton Hicks' "practice" contractions. For some, these increase in frequency up to the birth, while others feel very little.

There's your baby

The top of your uterus is around 6 in (15 cm) above your belly button by the end of this month. Your doctor can estimate your baby's size now by palpating your belly.

Forward planning

Having a baby forces you to reevaluate your home setup. Will you need a bigger, family-friendly car? Can you extend your home, or will you need to move in the near future? And what about your child's education, not to mention whether you've written a will? Phew! All that planning may leave you reeling slightly, but thinking about these things now can alleviate some pressure later on.

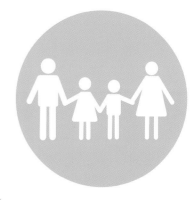

> Your blood volume peaks now at about 9 pints (5 liters). This dilutes red blood cells, so an iron-rich diet is important.

5 liters

By week 35
Your uterus will be about the size of a honeydew melon.

 At week 8   At week 12   At week 16

0 (cm)   10   20

Your growing baby

✳ Your baby's liver is now processing some waste and his kidneys are fully developed. He's preparing for life outside the uterus.

✳ Most babies begin to turn into their birth position about now—ideally with the head facing down.

✳ He has a rudimentary immune system in place, although he will rely upon the antibodies he receives through the umbilical cord and, later on, from breast milk, for some time to come.

✳ His eyes now open when he's awake, and close when he sleeps.

✳ Your uterus is becoming thinner as it stretches, allowing more light and sounds into his home.

✳ The average baby will gain about 1 lb (500 g) per week until birth.

✳ He will be quieter now, but will still have bursts of regular activity.

✳ Babies practice their facial expressions in response to external stimuli and even how they are feeling. They may grimace, frown, and even appear to smile while dreaming.

{ **Your baby** doesn't have much room now, and his movements will become slower and much more graceful. }

This month, think about...

● **Your hospital bag**
In addition to clothes and diapers for your baby, and your items, you may want to pack a camera; items to personalize your room or bed, such as your own pillows (check what the hospital allows); your cell phone (and charger) or change for pay phones; a list of people to contact after the birth; old or disposable underwear for post-birth lochia (bleeding); and something to wear home.

● **Ready for feeding**
Did you bring a comfortable nursing bra—one of the most important items for after the birth; or, if bottle-feeding, all the equipment you need?

● **Finer details**
Double-check the route to the hospital, and alternative ones in case of diversions or traffic, where you'll park, and make your plans for older children.

● **Stock up**
Now's the ideal time to get on the apron and batch-cook some meals to freeze, and stock up on pantry basics.

At week 21

At week 26

At week 30

By the end of this month, your baby measures **18 in** (46 cm) crown to heel.

30   40   50

The *nesting instinct*

We've all heard of nesting during pregnancy, but what exactly is the nesting instinct, and who has it?

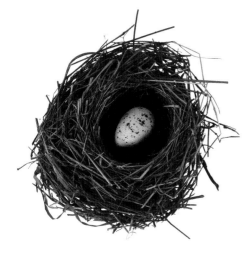

Even the least domestic of women can be driven to crazy bouts of cleaning and decorating during pregnancy. At this hormonally charged time, don't be surprised if you suddenly find yourself frantically scouring inside the oven, taking a toothbrush to bathroom tiles, color-coding clothes, or relentlessly stalking the aisles of 24-hour home stores in search of the perfect shade of baby-blue paint.

This maternal "nesting" impulse links us, spookily perhaps, to many species in the animal kingdom, but in particular to mammals that give birth to "immature" infants—those who can't immediately stand or follow their mother. Such mothers-to-be seek out a **safe place** well in advance, in order to birth and feed their newborn offspring comfortably. For example, cats and dogs gather soft items for warmth, field mice shred and weave grasses, and birds choose sites camouflaged or sheltered from adverse weather in order to successfully protect their nestlings.

Mother rabbits tear out their own fur to line their nests.

The amount of care mother animals put into nest building directly correlates to the amount and length of nurturing a newborn needs before it can live independently. This gives us humans license to go to town then, since our homes usually nurture our tiny tots well into their late teens (and often beyond). No wonder we feel so compelled to nest.

It is the increased levels of pregnancy hormones that trigger the onset of this maternal behavior, in particular oxytocin, the brain chemical associated with maternal bonding, and prolactin, the **"nesting hormone."** It's not just mothers-to-be who are affected—the nesting drive has been known to affect prospective adoptive mothers and even some men living with pregnant partners. It is therefore difficult to establish "instinctive" reactions in humans, given that our instincts are so over-layered with learned behavior and emotional responses. For this reason, many researchers refer to nesting as an "intuitive response" not an "instinct."

In a study conducted in 2011, 56 percent of expectant fathers experienced increased nesting activities.

So, what role does nesting play in pregnancy? In animals, an inadequate nesting area has been associated with failure of the young to thrive and reduced maternal responsiveness. For humans, nesting seems to allow women to exert some **control, calmness, and order** over what can seem an increasingly uncontrolled, stressful, and disordered life. Even as your expanding body demonstrates just how little control you have over pregnancy and the birth process, still you can build around you a place in which you feel psychologically and **emotionally safe**, creating an ambience that will equip you to cope with giving birth and taking care of a new baby. How reassuring to have everything clear and clean when a world of mess is rapidly approaching.

Establishing a sense of being safe and in control is valued by many midwives and natural-birth advocates as a key component for supporting a good labor—stress hormones, such as adrenaline, suppress the release of the hormone oxytocin, which promotes contractions. A study of pregnant women in Athens found that those who contemplated giving birth in the **familiar surroundings** of home had a sense of reassurance and safety that enhanced their self-esteem, and in turn boosted their confidence during labor.

Many birthing centers have adopted homey décor and deliberately non-medical protocols in a bid to make the most of our "human expression of nesting," counteracting some of the stress of labor and reducing feelings of risk.

Until parenthood arrives, life for most people involves commuting, working, and socializing. Yet when a new baby is imminent, this world starts to fade away. The gradual immobility of pregnancy and the drive to nest encourages a mother-to-be to spend more time at home connecting with neighbors and forming links with a local community. This perhaps reveals more shared animal characteristics—whether we are lions or humans, our young are easier to protect and more **likely to thrive** when enveloped in a larger social group. In evolutionary terms, this shift in behavior as we move toward the new role of parent reveals how successfully we adapt to changing circumstances.

When does the drive to nest strike? Most commonly from the fifth month of pregnancy, often accompanied by a spurt of energy. Take advantage by getting on top of tasks that require energy and enthusiasm—take a trip to the recycling center, **take time to shop** for the right stroller, and tie up loose ends on work projects. And if you feel compelled to do some of that house renovation work that's been hanging over you, make sure you use your common sense when it comes to the lifting and climbing—jobs such as these are best left to someone else at this stage.

By the end of the third trimester, the impulse to nest can go into **overdrive**. This is a well-documented sign of imminent labor, so if, in the days before your due date, you can't stop yourself from reaching for the drill or refolding baby clothes for the hundredth time, you may only have hours to go. Consider calling your doctor, who will use emotional and psychological—as well as physical—cues to diagnose labor's onset. Then prepare something sustaining to eat and take a nap before the real work of labor kicks in.

baby basics

Buying those first tiny outfits for your unborn child is one of life's great pleasures. Remember, though, to balance indulgence with practicality.

Historically, baby clothes (a "layette") would have been hand sewn during pregnancy and kept in a bottom drawer. These days, retail outlets are practically groaning with hundreds of different baby clothes, but how do you decide what to buy? Keep it simple—in the early weeks you are going to have enough on your plate without worrying about fancy outfits for your baby. The basic idea is to have enough layers and changes of outfit to deal with the weather and leaky diapers without having to do the laundry every day. That said, choosing these first outfits is one of the great joys of pregnancy—and amidst the baby basics, you can definitely indulge in some fabulously cute outfits, too.

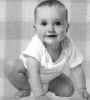

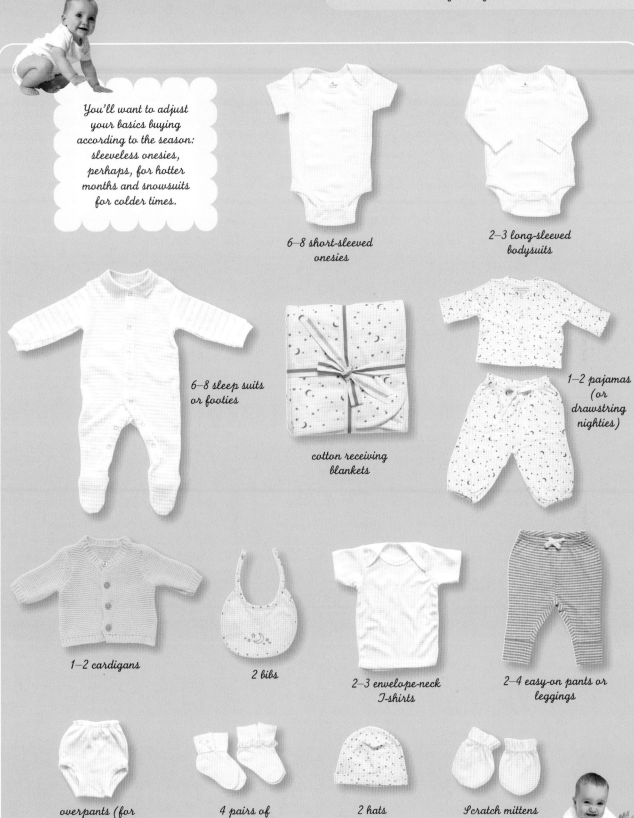

You'll want to adjust your basics buying according to the season: sleeveless onesies, perhaps, for hotter months and snowsuits for colder times.

6–8 short-sleeved onesies

2–3 long-sleeved bodysuits

6–8 sleep suits or footies

cotton receiving blankets

1–2 pajamas (or drawstring nighties)

1–2 cardigans

2 bibs

2–3 envelope-neck T-shirts

2–4 easy-on pants or leggings

overpants (for reuseable diapers)

4 pairs of socks

2 hats

Scratch mittens

Facts about
breast-feeding

Free, convenient, and available whenever required, your breast milk is the perfect first food for your baby. It provides all the nutrition and hydration she needs, and has numerous health benefits for you both.

What's in your milk?

Nutrient-rich colostrum gives way to transitional milk after five days, then to mature milk around day 15. Breast milk is almost 90 percent water, and contains around two hundred other components, including key nutrients, enzymes, hormones, growth factors, and antibodies. Breast milk adapts to meet your baby's needs: at the start of each feeding, the watery, low-fat "foremilk" is instantly thirst quenching; then the fat content rises as the creamy, calorie-rich "hindmilk" is released, making your baby full and content.

Super baby benefits

It's widely accepted that breast milk is best for babies. In addition to providing a sweet taste to attract your baby and a high nutritional value, breast milk will also boost your baby's immunity since it passes on disease-fighting antibodies and white blood cells. Research-based studies point to long-term protection against certain conditions, such as diabetes, heart disease, and childhood obesity. Breast-fed babies reportedly have fewer ear infections, stomach upsets, and respiratory complaints, and are more resistant to allergic conditions, such as eczema. Some studies even indicate that breast-fed children may have higher IQs.

Good for mom, too

There are some pretty convincing arguments on why breast-feeding is great for moms. After birth, your baby's sucking triggers the release of oxytocin, helping the uterus contract back to its usual size. Many women say that they lose weight breast-feeding, and research shows that it uses an extra 500 calories a day. Health benefits are impressive, too, with a lower incidence of postpartum depression and a reduced risk of breast, ovarian, and endometrial cancers in later life. And, contrary to old wives' tales, breast-feeding is good for your bone health, reducing your risk of developing osteoporosis.

WHAT DO YOU NEED?

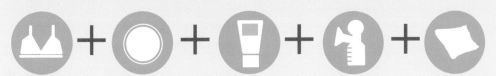

NURSING BRAS
A couple of fitted, supportive nursing bras will enable you to feed discreetly.

BREAST PADS
These are easily slipped inside your bra to absorb any small leaks.

NIPPLE CREAM
Sore or cracked nipples are soothed with a lanolin-based nipple cream.

BREAST PUMP
This can ease engorged breasts and enable you to bottle-feed.

BURP CLOTHS
Excellent for mopping up drooled milk, or draping over your nursing baby.

Breast-feeding facts

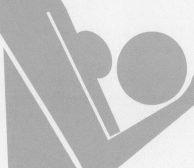

GLOBAL TRENDS

In the UK, 8 out of 10 women breast-feed at birth, up from 6 out of 10 in 1990.

Rwanda, Madagascar, and China have among the highest rates of women who breast-feed; they carry babies in slings, usually skin-to-skin.

In Canada, Norway, and Sweden, over 90 percent of mothers start breast-feeding.

DID YOU KNOW?

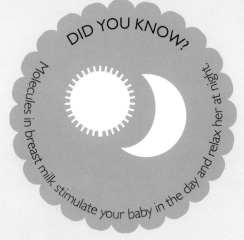

Molecules in breast milk stimulate your baby in the day and relax her at night.

Up to 75 percent of women produce more milk from their right breast.

IMMUNITY

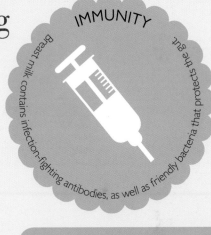

Breast milk contains infection-fighting antibodies, as well as friendly bacteria that protects the gut.

REALITY **CHECK**

 Too sore!
Your nipples need time to adjust to the sucking action, so keep in mind they might be sore while you're getting the hang of breast-feeding. If your baby has latched on properly it shouldn't be painful, so seek advice if necessary.

 Not so simple
Although heralded as the most natural thing in the world, breast-feeding can be difficult. Up to 75 percent of women seek help in the first few weeks, so don't feel alone if you are struggling. Talk to your doctor or pediatrician or a breast-feeding specialist and seek out a support group for more advice.

Facts about
formula-feeding

Breast-feeding isn't everyone's first choice. Discomfort or a medical condition are just two reasons why formula may be favored. If you choose formula, your baby will receive a high-quality, nutritious alternative to breast milk designed to meet his growing needs.

What's in formula?

Derived from cow's milk, formula is designed to give a baby optimum nutrition. It contains a complex mix of energy-providing nutrients in the form of carbohydrates, proteins, unsaturated fats, and added vitamins and minerals. Some have extras, such as omega-3 fatty acids to optimize development of the brain and nervous system, or pre- and probiotics for a healthy gut. Yet, many components of breast milk can't be replicated, such as the antibodies and the fat-digesting enzyme lipase—the lack of which makes formula harder to digest.

Benefits for baby

If you have chosen to go with formula, your baby will receive the key nutrients for healthy growth, including controlled amounts of vitamins and minerals, which avoids the need for supplements. If the formula is made up precisely as per the instructions, babies should gain weight at a steady, predictable pace. There are many different types of formula available so you can choose the one that best suits the needs of your baby. Parents confident in their choice of formula provide a relaxed feeding environment for their baby, and, crucially, bottle-feeding means that babies can experience a close feeding bond with Dad, too.

Good for parents, too

Being able to see exactly how much food your baby is getting is comforting—although weight gain provides extra reassurance. It's great for both parents to share the incredible feeling of nourishing their baby. Holding him close, even skin-to-skin, during feedings gives ample opportunity for bonding. Taking turns with nighttime feedings can be a godsend, and moms undeniably have greater freedom. Feedings tend to be less frequent since formula takes longer to digest than breast milk. What's more, moms don't face the prospect of painful nipples, or the worry about whether what they eat or drink will affect their baby.

WHAT DO YOU NEED?

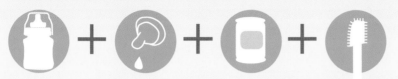

Six to eight bottles. Varying sizes allow the bottle to match your baby's appetite, but this is not strictly necessary.

Several nipples with different sized holes. Slow-flow nipples suit newborns; faster-flow suit older babies.

Baby formula. This needs to be mixed with cooled, boiled water according to the instructions.

Bottle brushes and cleaning equipment—it is essential to remove harmful bacteria.

DAILY AMOUNT

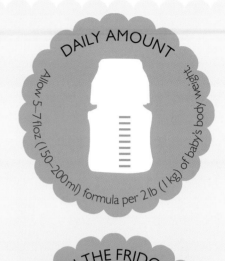

Allow 5–7 floz (150–200ml) formula per 2 lb (1 kg) of baby's body weight.

GLOBAL TRENDS

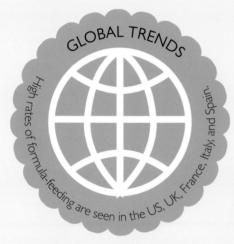

High rates of formula-feeding are seen in the US, UK, France, Italy, and Spain.

Higher rates of bottle-feeding occur in lower socioeconomic groups because women are less aware of breast-feeding benefits.

IN THE FRIDGE

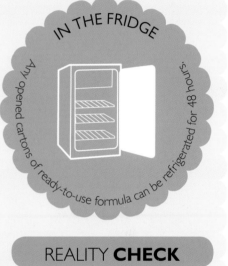

Any opened cartons of ready-to-use formula can be refrigerated for 48 hours.

Formula facts

Formulas with more "whey" protein in them are closer to breast milk and easier for a baby to digest.

DID YOU KNOW?

Bottle-feeding may benefit your love life! Lactation hormones may cause vaginal dryness, which can make lovemaking more challenging for breast-feeding moms.

The stools of formula-fed babies are the consistency of peanut butter.

REALITY **CHECK**

✓ *Time consuming*
All your equipment must be cleaned, dried, and the powder and water measured accurately.

✓ *Organization*
Adequate supplies are vital in case an extra feeding is needed.

✓ *A pricey business*
There's an ongoing financial cost.

✓ *Tummy troubles*
Formula can't match the complex benefits of breast milk, and since it is less easily digested formula can lead to stomach upsets.

Month 9

All about you

Room to breathe
Your baby drops deeper into your pelvic cavity this month, known aptly as "lightening" because of the easing of pressure on your diaphragm and ribs that suddenly makes breathing much easier. Of course, the pressure moves elsewhere and your baby now presses on your bladder.

Primed for production
Your breasts may be more tender as hormones produced by the placenta prepare them for feeding. You may leak some colostrum, your baby's "first" milk.

Take a seat
Don't feel guilty about putting your feet up more now. You're not slacking off, just very sensibly conserving energy for the big day.

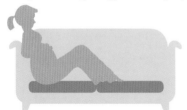

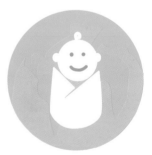

Nesting instinct
When you're not resting, you may be just itching to clean the house from top to bottom. The "nesting instinct" is a well-documented phenomenon, and while there's no harm succumbing to this urge, it's probably best to resist overdoing it.

Still growing
By week 40, your uterus has increased to about five times its normal size: in height from 3 in (7.5 cm) to 11¾ in (30 cm); in width from 2 in (5 cm) to 9 in (23 cm); and in depth 1 in (2.5 cm) to 7⅞ in (20 cm). Wow!

Forward planning
These last few weeks can feel like a bit of an emotional roller coaster as you wait for labor, caught between anxiety and excitement. Time is also taken up ensuring that everything is in place. In the midst of all this, it can be easy to lose focus of the main point—that you're about to become parents. When you get the chance, it's worth spending some time just stopping and reflecting on this incredible and often hard-to-process fact: how your world is about to change when you welcome your baby into your lives. A little scary, yes, but extraordinarily wonderful too!

Keeping active will help encourage the contractions that will bring your baby into the world.

By week 40
Your uterus will be about the size of a watermelon.

Your growing baby

* By 37 weeks, your baby is "clinically mature." She has an excellent chance of surviving outside the uterus with little or no support.

* Your baby will continue to put on weight until she is born; the average baby weighs between 5½lb (2.5 kg) and 8¾lb (4 kg) at term.

* As her head settles into your pelvic cavity, she will be able to stretch her legs a little more.

* Your baby has more than 70 different reflexes—or instinctive, involuntary, and almost instantaneous reactions to certain stimuli—that are designed to protect her and ensure her survival.

* She practices for life outside the uterus by sucking, or "breathing," amniotic fluid, urinating, and sleeping.

* Her face is filling out and she has recognizable eyelashes and a thicker neck, which is more in proportion to her head.

* Your baby's adrenal glands are about 20 times larger than an adult's to coordinate her growth and development and kick-start labor. They'll return to their natural size a couple of weeks after birth.

* The surge of maternal hormones before labor means that your baby's genitals appear swollen and out of proportion.

This month, think about...

Backup plans
Do you have someone you can call if your partner can't be with you right away on the day? However unlikely this scenario, it can be reassuring to know all eventualities are covered.

Dress rehearsal
Have you tried a trial run to the hospital during rush hour?

Child-care plans
Do you need to give older children a try-out staying with a relative or friend who will be taking care of them when you're giving birth, so that this is familiar and reassuring for them on the actual day?

Ready for labor
It may feel a bit silly, but have you practiced breathing techniques with your partner —you may both appreciate this preparation on the day; and spending some time trying out massage techniques is relaxing now, and potentially crucial for the imminent labor.

> *In the last weeks, your baby's heart rate gradually slows to around 120–160 beats per minute (bpm). A sudden drop signals the start of labor.*

120–160 bpm

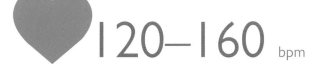

At week 21   At week 26   At week 30   At week 34   By the end of this month, your baby measures about **20½in** (52 cm) crown to heel.

30   40   50

What's in a *name?*

Carrying the weight of history, heritage, and hopes, choosing a name can seem fraught with difficulties.

All cultures place huge significance on the act of baby naming, and in many traditions, naming is itself a spiritual act. In creation stories from Christian to Hindu, and Aboriginal to Native American traditions, the world comes into being only when the unique name of an object is uttered out loud. The divine syllable "om" was the first sound and brought everything in the universe to life, say the Hindu scriptures. Aboriginal creation myths tell of birds, plants, animals, and rocks springing into being from nothingness as their names are sung. In the Pueblo tradition, the mythical figure, Thought Woman, imagines everything in the universe, but nothing exists until she gives each object its name. A **name empowers us with identity** and connects past, present, and future.

So which name will you choose? Maybe you will dip into your **hereditary pool**, rich with references formulated over generations. In parts of Ghana, to bestow the name of lost loved ones brings those ancestors back to life, sowing the seeds of their attributes in a new tiny being. In other places, family names reveal a child's background: his line of descent, social standing, and family position. Balinese tradition locks a child's gender, caste, clan, and birth order into four names before giving a fifth "personal" name.

Despite having an intensely personal meaning, a name is a very public thing.

Grandparents and grandchildren are often yoked together by a name; for example, in England it has been common since the 1700s to name a first son after his father's father and a second son after his mother's father. The Edu people in Nigeria honor grandfathers and great-grandfathers by having them officiate at naming ceremonies or choose the name. Elsewhere, too, the choice of name is out of parents' hands. Sikh families attend a ceremony at their gurdwara where a page is picked at random from the holy book as a prayer is said. The first letter of the first word on the left-hand page gives the first letter of the baby's name.

> In China, each of the five elements: metal, wood, water, fire, and earth, are represented in a name by a character or a word with the qualities of that element.

In many cultures, a name is thought to **influence a child's future life chances, behavior, and accomplishments**. In China, the number of strokes in a written name is said to determine the child's fate. While in early New England, virtues were handed to daughters—Patience, Prudence, Charity—and in Victorian Britain, names of illustrious or noble people were popular, hence the many Victorias, Alberts, and Clives. Auspicious names with an amuletic quality, such as Lucky, that augur well and offer protection from ill-wishers are common in parts of Africa. Sometimes they deflect evil by invoking laughter.

For Islamic parents, **a name is a thing of beauty**, denoting an honorable quality, innate goodness, or devotion to God. Jameela, for example, means "good character" and "beautiful." Christians might choose the name of a **saint for whom they feel an affinity** or whose feast day is near the birth. The Yoruba people believe each name has a **spirit that lives through a child** regardless of his nature. This chimes with parents who wait before giving a name until a child shows him-or herself—through looks, demeanor, or spirit—to be a Ruby, Rufus, or an Apple.

Made-up names reflecting **topicality and celebrity culture** are big in some parts of the world, for example, Briella, a US hit in 2011—though daughters are more often recipients then sons. Boys' names tend to remain stable. William has been in the top 20 US names for over a century, although there are changing trends: once neglected Old Testament figures such as Jacob, Elijah, and Noah have enjoyed a surge in popularity recently, challenging previously popular New Testament names such as Matthew, Mark, and Luke, more commonplace in the 20th century.

In some countries, parents select from a **state-approved list**. Denmark's Law on Personal Names gives 7,000 standard names. Parents can seek permission for another name through the church, and the case is investigated by officials.

Sometimes a name arrives at birth. Eskimo birth attendants recite names as the child is pushed out: the infant "chooses" his name by appearing when called. Luo babies in Kenya stop crying when "their" name is recited. In Ghana, a child takes a temporary "birth" name of the day of the week; and the elements of a Chinese name can reflect the hour, day, month, and year, connecting an infant with his horoscope.

A **naming ceremony** offers families a chance to gather and renew ties. Regardless of spiritual heritage, this is a time for new beginnings and hope. Some parents create custom ceremonies, appropriating customs from different traditions and starting new ones. In a "baby-wish whisper," each person whispers to the baby what they would wish her to take through life: a loving disposition, appreciation of music, gentleness, and so on. Attendees may give a personal name, as is common in Nigeria and Ghana, or chant a song with the name, as in Hindu naming ceremonies, or for the Saami people, blessed by parents with a "joik" or "acoustic symbol" personal to their life. Sharing a feast, giving a name, and wishing a child health, long life, and prosperity, entwines lives and enfolds the new babe into family and community.

Facts about
natural pain relief

If you are averse to taking drugs during labor, you may worry that your pain relief options will be limited. But, rest assured there is a good selection of natural therapies available with real benefits and no side effects—from techniques you can practice at home, to treatments that you can take with you to ease your pain.

What are the options?

Massage
Soothing massage stimulates the release of endorphins, your body's natural painkiller, helping to promote relaxation. Your partner can try out techniques before labor. Lower back and buttock pain responds to firm, deep pressure. Between contractions, a therapeutic shoulder massage can release tension. Communication is key: tell your partner exactly what you need, keeping in mind that on the day it may be different.

Hypnobirthing
This "complete" birthing program combines relaxation with visualization and simple self-hypnosis. It aims to help you release fear and enter a state of deep relaxation during labor, so that you can welcome the "surge" of each contraction that brings your baby closer. Studies indicate that women who practice hypnobirthing have shorter labor times, fewer medical interventions, and less need of drugs.

Breathing techniques
Releasing slow, steady breaths during contractions is a great way to focus the mind and relieve tension—the intake of breath will be a natural reflex for your body, so concentrate on your out-breath. Holding your breath in response to pain (a natural instinct) impedes oxygen flow and tenses up your muscles; practicing rhythmic breathing before labor teaches you to focus on your breath.

Applying heat relaxes muscles and stimulates blood flow.

GLOBAL TRENDS

Water births and hypnobirthing have become increasingly popular.

BIRTH PARTNER

If you have a hospital birth, your birth partner will be able to see the peaks and valleys of your contractions via a monitor. By telling you once you are over the worst part, they can help you manage your pain during each contraction.

Birth partners can help with breathing, massage, or helping you into a pool.

The facts

REALITY **CHECK**

✓ **Medical necessity**
You may choose to avoid drugs if you can help it, preferring to feel every moment of your birth experience. But remember labor is unpredictable—be prepared in case you need intervention, such as an induction or an emergency C-section.

✓ *Give me the drugs!*
Don't be stoical if you find the pain is too much. Brush up on what drugs are available so you can choose, if you need to (see pages 102–103).

TENS machine
A TENS (transcutaneous electrical nerve stimulation) machine is a device that transmits electrical impulses believed to block pain signals from reaching the brain. Wires from the TENS machine attach to pads on your back. Its effectiveness is best suited to early labor, it has no known side effects, and leaves you free to move around. Although widely used in the UK, TENS machines are less commonly used in the US.

Water births
Warm water is excellent for laboring—it has a soothing effect on your muscles and helps you to relax, while the natural buoyancy supports your body taking pressure off the spine and pelvis. This means you can move more freely without getting too tired. You also enjoy one-on-one care, since you will not be left in the pool unattended. Birthing pools are available in some birthing centers and increasingly in hospitals—you can also rent (or buy) one for use at home.

In your home, you can get in the pool whenever you like, but in the hospital you will probably have to wait until labor is well established, or once your cervix is 5 cm dilated. There is no evidence to suggest that there is an increased risk of infection by giving birth in water, and your baby's innate "dive" reflex stops him from inhaling on contact with the water. Water temperature is kept at a maximum of 99.5°F (37.5°C) to prevent you from overheating and distressing your baby.

Facts about
medical pain relief

Dealing with labor pains is a common source of worry. Various drugs are available that can help ease your birth experience.

What are the options?

Opioids

This class of drugs—which are narcotics, including morphine—block the transmission of pain in the body by attaching themselves to receptors in the brain or nerves. During labor, opioids help some women relax, allowing them to have a more positive experience. Other women experience nausea or dizziness when they're given opioids, which detracts from the experience. Opioids cross the placenta and can sedate your baby or affect her breathing, so they shouldn't be given too close to delivery time.

Tranquilizers

This class of drugs is not intended to relieve pain directly, but they can relieve anxiety in women who are extremely fearful or anxious about experiencing labor and delivery. Women who use tranquilizers during labor don't recall the experience fully, because the drug makes them feel sleepy and disoriented, although it can help an anxious person get through the experience. The drug crosses the placenta, making the baby sluggish.

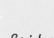 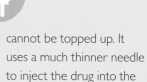

Epidural

A local anesthetic is injected into the space between the membrane covering the spinal cord and the bony spinal column in the lower back (known as the epidural space). This anesthetic gives complete pain relief, numbing the lower part of your body but leaving you awake and alert. It acts within 20 minutes and can be "topped up" throughout labor, as necessary.

Spinal block

This is another local anesthetic to the lower back. Like an epidural it provides complete relief in the lower body, but is a "one time shot" only and cannot be topped up. It uses a much thinner needle to inject the drug into the sac of spinal fluid below the spinal cord. The pain relief kicks in within minutes, but lasts only an hour or two.

Combined spinal–epidural block

A combined spinal–epidural block may give the best of both worlds—it offers the speedy pain relief of the spinal block alongisde the ongoing top-up option of the epidural.

:(POSSIBLE SIDE EFFECTS

Tranquilizers	Opioids	Epidural		Spinal block
Can make you feel distant, disoriented, confused, or sleepy. Does not directly affect pain levels.	Can make you sleepy, nauseous, and can't be given close to delivery since they may slow the baby's breathing and heart rate.	Can prolong the pushing part of labor and prevent you from feeling your contractions, so you will have to be told when to push by medical staff.	Your legs may feel heavy, you may need a catheter to urinate, have backache for a day or two, and, in rare instances, a headache.	Can cause your blood pressure to decrease, which can slow the baby's heart rate.

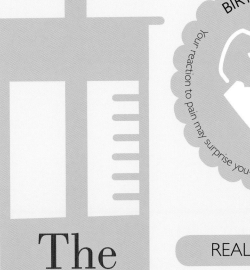

The facts

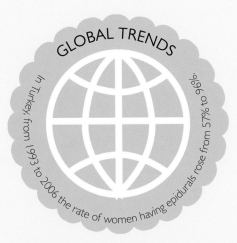

GLOBAL TRENDS

In Turkey, from 1993 to 2006 the rate of women having epidurals rose from 57% to 66%

In the US, epidurals are the primary form of pain relief during labor.

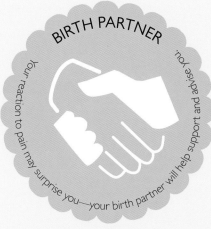

BIRTH PARTNER

Your reaction to pain may surprise you—your birth partner will help support and advise you.

REALITY **CHECK**

✓ *Medical necessity*
It's good to be informed about your pain relief options. Some women feel more divorced from the birth process by using medical pain relief, and find drug-free births empowering. Conversely, others feel more in control of their bodies and birth if they have made an informed choice to opt for, say, an epidural.

DID YOU KNOW?

Epidurals are administered by an anesthesiologist; if yours is busy you may now have to wait.

Endorphins are opiatelike brain chemicals that are naturally released by the body in response to pain.

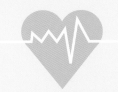

Facts about *Cesareans*

Having your baby by cesarean is increasingly common in the developed world—in Western Europe about one in every four to five babies are delivered this way. Cesareans are either planned or performed in an emergency situation, and can be life saving for both mother and child. Although routinely done, a cesarean is, nevertheless, an invasive surgical procedure that requires recovery time.

What is a Cesarean?

A cesarean (or C-section) is an operation to cut through your abdomen and then your uterus to reach your baby and take him out. The cut is usually made through the bikini line (transverse cut)—though it can also be done vertically—and it is then sewn up immediately afterward.

What will happen?

Your pubic area will be shaved and a catheter linked to your bladder. You will be hooked up to an intravenous line to provide fluid and medication. Usually a local anesthetic will be given to numb the lower part of your body, leaving you awake for your baby's birth. A screen may be placed across you, behind which the surgeon cuts through your abdomen and uterus to take out your baby and then the placenta. While you hold your new baby you will be stitched up. The whole procedure should take about 30–45 minutes.

Why you might need one

A cesarean is called elective if it is planned ahead of your due date. This may happen if your baby is in a difficult position to deliver vaginally (for example, breech), you are carrying twins or more, your placenta is covering the opening of your cervix, or if there are other medical risks to you or your baby. However, you may start labor naturally but need an emergency cesarean. This may happen if there are risks to you or your baby by continuing, for example if your baby becomes distressed, or he shows an abnormal heartbeat, or if your labor is not progressing.

☹ POSSIBLE RISKS

Risks to the mother

These include infection, excess blood loss, blood clots, and accidental damage to the bladder, ovaries, and uterus.

Risks to the baby

About 35 out of 1,000 babies born by cesarean will have breathing problems after birth, compared with just 5 of every 1,000 born vaginally.

BOND WITH BABY

You should be able to immediately cuddle and breast-feed your baby.

GIVING BIRTH AGAIN

Women were once told "once a cesarean always a cesarean": this is no longer the case. Discuss the risks of a normal birth versus a second C-section with your doctor.

The chances of a successful normal birth after cesarean are up to 76 percent.

Successful cesareans have saved the lives of countless women and babies worldwide

RECOVERY TIME

6 weeks

You may be out of bed hours after surgery, but full recovery time is about six weeks.

Cesarean facts

In the US, a fear of malpractice suits may influence doctors to recommend cesareans.

GLOBAL TRENDS

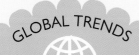

18.5 million

babies annually are born by cesarean. Brazil and China boast the world's highest rates, with almost one in two babies born by cesarean; in the US one in three babies are born this way.

Increasing rates of older moms, obesity, and multiple births mean rising rates of cesareans.

REALITY **CHECK**

✓ *Invasive*
It may take a while to get back to normal—surgery is traumatic and you need time to heal.

✓ *Stuck at home*
Not being able to drive for six weeks can be challenging; check your car insurance details, too.

✓ *Let down*
Some women can feel cheated out of their birth experience by a cesarean. But once you're holding your beautiful new baby, how he got there doesn't matter.

Bring *it on*

Women through the ages have tried a range of ways to bring on labor when they are overdue. Whether you're trying to avoid an induction, your pelvis is complaining, or you're just impatient to meet your little one, you may want to give nature a helping hand.

Eat your greens

"Labor salads" becoming popular, where restaurants come up with their own labor-inducing recipes. A typical one consists of equal parts of Romaine lettuce, watercress, and red cabbage, with a balsamic vinaigrette. The balsamic is said to be the key although there's no evidence why. Should taste good though.

Get the point

Some people swear by acupuncture to start labor when you are very overdue. This ancient Chinese art involves the insertion of tiny needles into specific points in your body and is thought to stimulate the body's energy to act on specific organs or systems.

Aah, a nice cup of tea

Thought to strengthen the muscles of the uterus, drinking raspberry leaf tea may pique your curiosity, but don't try this herbal product until your baby is full-term (37 weeks), in case it causes labor. Herbal products are generally not recommended during pregnancy.

Oh-so sexy

Orgasm can trigger the release of oxytocin, the hormone that starts and regulates your contractions. If you can't face full-fledged sex when you are overdue, a bit of nipple stimulation is a less energetic option! The idea is to trick your body into thinking you're breast-feeding, causing your uterus to contract.

Get up off the sofa

Mild exercise, such as a brisk walk or housecleaning, can sometimes be all you need to get things going, since the weight of your baby's head on your pelvis may help prime your cervix. Other suggestions are bouncing on a birthing ball or driving on a bumpy road.

Spice things up

The theory is that hot spices, for example those found in a curry, can stimulate your stomach and bowel muscles, especially if you're not used to spicy foods. This muscle stimulation has a secondary effect on the uterine muscles, kick-starting contractions.

Titillate

Stimulating your nipples naturally releases oxytocin, which can trigger contractions. To best mimic the sucking action of a baby, massage the surrounding areola as well as the nipple itself.

Activate

Stimulating the muscles of your digestive system, for example through eating curry or taking castor oil, could result in the stimulation of the muscles of your uterus.

Squeeze

An orgasm releases oxytocin and causes the muscles of the uterus and vagina to contract. The point is to propel sperm toward the fallopian tubes, but it may also kick-start labor!

Soften

Semen contains hormonelike substances called prostaglandins. These help to relax smooth muscle, and, if deposited near the cervix during sex, can encourage it to soften and dilate.

DID YOU KNOW?

Oxytocin is also called the love hormone: it plays a key role in orgasm, labor, and breast-feeding, and is also believed to help couples to form a stable bond after having sex.

No natural means of inducing labor will work if your body is not ready!

The uterus "practices" for labor during pregnancy—these tightenings are called Braxton Hicks' contractions

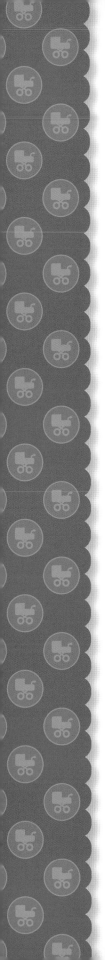

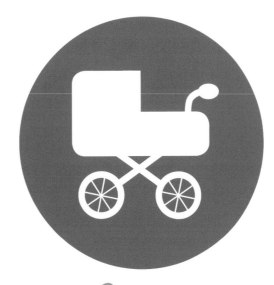

Deep *breaths*

Pregnancy and birth
around the world

More than 350,000 babies are born every day. Discover how different cultures embrace the unique wonder of birth.

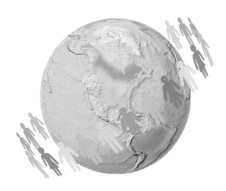

There are thousands of wonderfully diverse cultures around the world, separated by differences in language, religion, philosophy, and perspective. However, there is one thing that unifies them— the single act of giving birth and bringing new life into this world. And while attitudes and customs surrounding pregnancy and childbirth differ wildly across the globe, there is no doubt that there is a huge amount to be learned from each other's **knowledge and experience**.

All women feel an increased need to protect themselves (and their growing baby) during pregnancy, by trying to **avoid stress and guard against unnecessary risk**. Yet the lengths to which different women will go to achieve this vary hugely. Some women in Central America, particularly those of Mayan descent, are so fearful of exposure to disease, evil spirits, and even the ill will of others that they may spend the whole nine months at home. In some Asian countries, it is strongly believed that a woman's mental state during her pregnancy can **influence the personality of the unborn child**, and so pregnant women avoid funerals, sex, fits of temper, and even gossiping. At the other end of the spectrum there are many women, such as those in Ethiopia, who find it more reassuring to view pregnancy as a **natural part of life** so they don't make many changes in their daily routine.

Giving birth is a primal and instinctive act, but in many countries it is also governed by **ancient customs** intended to facilitate the process. Indian mothers, for instance, wear their hair down and remove jewelry and head coverings in order to abandon constraint and **embrace the natural process of labor**; all doors and windows in the house are opened to symbolically encourage an easy passage for the baby. In Morocco, women are treated to tummy rubs with oil and herbal infusions to alleviate pain. Guatemalan women drink beer in which a purple onion has been boiled in order to speed up delivery, while some Native Americans use blue cohosh root, because it is believed to encourage uterine contractions. In some cultures, birth is considered to be highly sacred. For example, while the **placenta and umbilical cord** are often regarded as mere by-products of birth, in many communities they are viewed as potent forces, with the power to influence the baby's future. In Japan, the umbilical cord is cleaned and put in a special box in the belief that it will promote a **strong mother–child relationship**. In Mali, the placenta is believed to be closely connected to the baby's welfare, and after the birth is cleaned and placed in a basket that the baby's father will then bury.

In Syria, mothers are prescribed parsley to help bring their milk in, while some Indian women bathe in cows' milk after baby is born.

The period immediately after birth is one of transition, and most women are heavily supported during this time. Many cultures even impose a traditional **confinement period**. In Italy and Colombia, mother and baby are expected to stay in the house for 40 days to avoid exposure to the cold and to germs. This is echoed in China where new mothers are protected from wind and even cold drafts from air-conditioning units and fans, since exposure is believed to weaken the body, leaving it susceptible to illness. In Vietnam, the **mother-in-law** moves in for a month to take charge of preparing hearty soups and stews containing medicinal ingredients, such as ginger and sesame (both associated with maternal health). To many parents, this level of constant care may seem an unwelcome intrusion, since time alone with the baby or as a new family unit would be

On the third day of a Tibetan baby's life, people bring gifts of yak-butter tea, barley wine, and cheese to represent wishes for an abundant life.

limited, and the freedom to make mistakes and learn the ropes on their own is something many new parents crave. However, few people could complain about the arrangements in the Netherlands, where **every new mother is provided with a maternity nurse** who visits the baby at home for several hours on each of the first ten days. Equally appealing is the Indonesian tradition, where new mothers are given **daily 90-minute massages** with a blend of special herbs, to soothe away aches and stress, and even reduce the risk of blood clots.

Every culture has its own unique way of **welcoming a new addition**, from the Balinese tradition of ensuring the baby's feet do not touch the ground for 105 days, to the Inuit custom of greeting a new baby with a handshake. But one thing that seems to be instinctive to us all, as humans, is for **family and friends to gather** to hold and meet the baby, in order to welcome her into their wider community.

Some **customs are echoed** again and again across the globe, with only small variations in the way they are practiced—indicating that there are just as many ideals and beliefs that unify us as there are those that set us apart. While some concepts are so unfamiliar that they may seem outlandish, there are few that do not have some sound basis in caring for infants and new mothers. Either way, babies are coming into this world successfully every day, and men and women are beginning parenthood in their own individual way—just as they have been doing for millennia in every part of our increasingly small world.

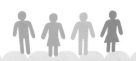

Facing the *fear*

Labor: the final frontier. The last hurdle to cuddling your new baby looms large, thanks to the uncertainty surrounding the timing, what will happen, and the worries about pain. Feeling optimistic, confident, calm, and well supported will help you better manage labor.

I'm scared of labor

Life experiences this dramatic are rare, so it's OK to feel daunted. Some women experience labor as a struggle for survival, whereas others view it as an empowering experience. It's hard to predict how your body will cope, particularly the first time, so get acquainted with all pain-relief options and be ready to adapt your birth plan.

How does labor start?

In the final weeks of pregnancy, hormones soften the cervix to prepare for labor. The onset of contractions is triggered by the release of the hormone oxytocin.

What happens next?

Vaginal birth is often split into **three stages**. In the first (the "latent stage"), the uterus starts contracting and the cervix thins and shortens, drawing up over the baby's head (effacement), before stretching and opening (dilatation). At the end of this stage the cervix is fully dilated and your contractions are strong, yet you lack the urge to push. This is the time when you might tell everyone that you have had enough and **want to go home**, but the labor nurses will interpret this as a positive sign that you are in "transition," and that **delivery is imminent**. During the second stage, intense contractions push the baby through the birth canal and out into the world. In the third and final stage, the placenta is delivered and the umbilical cord is cut.

How much will it hurt?

During contractions, pain is intense. Women in a 2005 study rated it on a scale of 6.7–9.6 out of 10. Ouch! Stress, anxiety, and feeling powerless can make any pain seem worse, so try to remember this pain is purposeful and that it will end. Each contraction brings your baby closer. Focus on the pain-free gaps between contractions and use pain relief if you need it.

What if I embarrass myself?

Women in labor scream, shout, swear, and soil themselves. Medical staff are not phased by this and have seen it all before. You'll be too busy to be embarrassed, and are unlikely to remember the details afterward.

I hate the idea of seeing my partner in pain

You're in good company. This is the reason men most often give for avoiding the delivery room, and it can lead to feelings of frustration and helplessness. Childbirth classes can help you feel prepared, and specific classes for dads-to-be explore common fears and reactions during labor. Being involved in the delivery of your child can help foster an earlier and more intense bond between father, mother, and baby.

How will I know how to help her?

Just be there. Trials show that continuous emotional support during labor significantly reduces cesarean sections and forceps deliveries, and lessens the need for pain relief. Familiarizing yourself with what to expect in the delivery room will be a big help. The more you know about childbirth, the better equipped you are to help, the happier your partner will be with your support, and the more positive everyone's experience will be. So, read up well beforehand.

Why do I have pains, too?

The transition to fatherhood can trigger physical and psychological symptoms, such as morning sickness, bloating, and insomnia, known as "couvade." The increased involvement of fathers at birth has seen a peak in "sympathetic pregnancy" and Italian research puts it at up to 65 percent of dads-to-be. Attending childbirth classes with your partner will help to alleviate the emotional, bonding, and stress issues that contribute to the phenomenon.

How can your *birth partner* help?

If you want a shorter, calmer, and happier labor, then find yourself a birth partner. Then, talk through everything so he or she is completely in the know.

Your birth partner could be your partner, mother, a doula (specialized labor coach), midwife, sibling, or close friend. Whoever you choose, your birth partner needs to be **reliable and calm**. The job description is to support you, communicate for you if needed, provide your basic needs such as drinks and snacks, **bolster your confidence,** and provide continuity as labor nurses change shifts. Ideally your birth partner should attend childbirth classes with you so he or she knows what to expect, and you can discuss ideas of what you'd like to happen well before the day. Emotional support is key. It's basic stuff—praising you, encouraging you, and reassuring you, and simply just being there with you. Your partner's comfort and support will help **reduce your anxiety and stress levels,** and even the physical pain you feel.

Having a birth partner is just as important if you are having a **cesarean**, whether planned or emergency. He or she can be with you in the operating room to talk to you and reassure you, and speak on your behalf to medical staff and anesthesiologists.

Your birth partner will also have an important role to play **after the birth** since you will have someone to talk to about how it went, and share in the happiness. Sometimes mothers (and fathers) feel that labor and birth did not live up to expectations or go according to plan. You will appreciate having someone to talk through your feelings with afterward, which **can help you feel positive** about your experience.

Partners, try these out...

✳ Help with breathing and relaxation techniques, get the birthing ball, help with the TENS machine, hold your partner in a comfortable position as labor progresses, and get in the birth pool if asked!

✳ Be a good distraction. Talk to her and read aloud from a book, newspaper, or magazine. Use humor to keep her spirits up, but also be sensitive to when she needs you to be quiet.

{ *Use the gentle massage techniques learned in childbirth classes and massage her lower back, hands, or feet, as directed. Help her to use the rests between contractions to stretch her muscles and change positions for comfort.* }

✳ Provide food and drinks for you both. She may be permitted to have clear beverages; ask the nurses first. Remember to take supplies with you to prevent lengthy trips away from the delivery room.

✳ *Play some of her favorite music to try to distract her or help her relax.*

✳ Meditate together during early labor to help her relax. Meditation can help block unnecessary noise and a busy environment.

✳ Be your partner's advocate. When she is too tired or in too much pain to fully communicate with doctors and nurses, be ready to ask for help, tell them her wishes, and ask for further explanations.

Positions for an easier *birth*

How you position yourself during labor can help you manage the pain and speed of delivery, and help your baby arrive as easily and quickly as possible. Your baby might need monitoring during your labor, but for much of the time an active, mobile labor should help you have an easier birth.

STRIKE A POSE

In one study, walking, sitting, and kneeling were shown to shorten the first stage by about an hour and reduce the need for epidural anesthesia by 17 percent, compared with lying down.

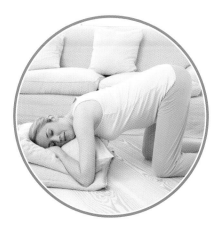

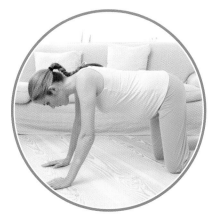

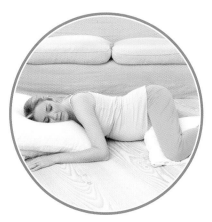

Lean forward

Whether standing or on your knees, leaning forward can alleviate pain in your lower back and allow you some well-earned rest, while keeping your pelvis in a helpful position. Try resting your forearms on the bed, sofa, cushions, or a sturdy cupboard—whatever you have on hand.

On all fours

Rocking forward and back on your hands and knees eases back pain and can make a welcome change from other positions. Cushion your feet and knees with rolled-up towels or a pillow. If your wrists hurt, kneel up and lean onto a pile of cushions, a birthing ball, or your partner.

On your side

If you want to lie in bed and rest during a long labor, try lying on one side (ideally left) with the opposite leg raised for pushing. This keeps the pelvic bones moving apart to allow the baby through the birth canal. Research also suggests that it's the best position for avoiding tears when pushing.

Throughout Asia, Africa, and the Americas squatting is a favored birth position.

Squatting

By allowing your pelvis to open fully, with the sacrum and coccyx moving back, squatting allows gravity to encourage your baby's movement downward. If you're not used to it, squatting can be tiring for your legs, so in the early stage of labor try sitting on a birthing ball, and in the second stage (when pushing), a birthing chair or stool. Pushing from an upright position is thought to shorten the second stage of labor and to reduce the need for an assisted delivery or episiotomy, but for some it might increase slightly the risk of second-degree tears and blood loss during pushing.

Not on your back

The least helpful position for giving birth is lying on your back: it reduces space in the pelvis and forces the baby to travel uphill, while the weight of the uterus and the baby can interfere with blood flow to the placenta. That said, lying on your back is the most common position for birth in health-care facilities worldwide. It might be because women like to rest on their backs at the end of labor or because it is the easiest position for your health-care team to monitor you and your baby. Even if you deliver on your back, try to spend as much of your early stage labor being up and around.

Moving around

Being upright expands the diameter of your pelvis slightly, reduces pressure on nerves in the spine, and allows gravity to help your baby through the birth canal. When you are upright and moving around, your baby's head engages with your cervix more directly and evenly, making contractions more efficient. Walk slowly, sway, and pace from foot to foot. Breathe consciously as you move to help you to relax, and to improve your circulation. Resist the urge to hold your breath and tighten your body when you experience a contraction.

Welcome to the *world*

Your baby is about to enter the big wide world, and at birth she will undergo some dramatic physical changes.

LIFE ON THE INSIDE

Take a breath

For nine months your baby has been safely ensconced in a watery world where she doesn't need to breathe. Oxygen is brought to her from your body via the umbilical cord and placenta, and carbon dioxide waste is transported away. During the last weeks in the uterus, her tiny, flattened lungs practice breathing in and out, but it is amniotic fluid, and not air, that flows through them.

Beating heart

Your baby's circulation follows a different route when she is in the uterus. Because she has no need to take oxygen into her lungs most of her blood flow bypasses them. Instead, oxygen-rich blood from the placenta travels from one side of the heart to the other via a small hole called the foramen ovale. Her circulating blood is propelled along by the beating of her heart, not yours.

Wrap me up

Your baby has been kept warm and snug in the uterus. At 99.7°F (37.6°C), the amniotic fluid cushioning her is just slightly warmer than your body temperature, and stays constant, whatever the temperature is outside.

I'm hungry...

Your baby has become accustomed to a never-ending stream of nutrients in the uterus, delivered to her from the placenta, via the umbilical cord.

Keeping safe

Your uterus is relatively sterile, so going out into the world will be an assault on your baby's immune system. Antibodies transfer across the placenta and into your baby's bloodstream via the umbilical cord, which will help to prepare his immune system ready for arrival.

I can see!

Your baby's eyelids were fused in the first trimester, but at about 28 weeks she opens her eyes for the first time. The layers of her retina have developed, including the light-sensitive rods and cones, so now she can distinguish light from dark—even through the abdominal wall.

It's noisy here

Hearing is one of the first senses to develop, and by 22 weeks her ears are almost completely formed. She may be able to hear and respond to your voice from 25 weeks.

IN THE REAL WORLD

Take a breath

Within seconds of birth, your baby will take her first breath—often giving her first reassuring cry with it—which opens up the airways. The lungs empty of fluid and each successive breath gradually gets easier.

Beating heart

With her first gasp of air, the circulation re-routes itself, now flowing from the right side of the heart to the lungs where it picks up oxygen and travels back to the left side of the heart to be pumped to the body. The foramen ovale should seal shut due to the pressure of returning blood from the lungs to the left side of the heart.

Wrap me up

Once she is born, your baby won't be able to regulate her own body temperature—she will lose heat easily but cannot shiver or rely on muscle movement to generate heat. Full-term babies are born with a tailor-made fuel supply of brown fat around their neck, upper chest, and kidneys. This is especially good at generating heat but it soon runs out, so keeping your baby warm after birth is a priority. Holding her close against your body as soon as she is born will help her to absorb your body warmth.

I'm hungry…

Being born is hard work for your baby, and she will have a powerful drive to look for nourishment soon after. Newborn babies have primitive reflexes that help them feed; the rooting reflex makes your baby turn her mouth toward you if you stroke her cheek, and the suckling reflex helps her to take milk from the breast or bottle. Your baby has a tiny tummy—the size of a walnut—and it may need to be filled every two hours at the beginning.

Keeping safe

Breast-feeding will provide your baby with a further supply of antibodies to help fight bugs she encounters in the world outside. She is also born with a waxy layer over her skin called vernix, which acts as a barrier to infection until it is absorbed by the body.

I can see!

Your baby may blink at bright lights when she is born. She can only see a distance of about 8–10 in (20–25 cm), just enough to look at your face when feeding and can see only in shades of light and dark; her color vision won't function until weeks after she is born. Her eyes may be puffy from squeezing through the birth canal.

It's noisy here

The outside world may seem like a cacophony to your baby who will get startled at loud noises, but remember inside your uterus was noisy, too. White noise, such as radio static, hair dryers, or vacuum cleaners, can soothe a newborn by mimicking the sounds heard in utero.

Your newborn's thymus gland is larger than an adult's—it produces white blood cells, helping to develop her immunity.

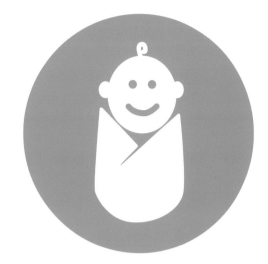

A mini *miracle*

First few *moments*

Nothing prepares you for the incredible moment when you finally meet your baby. At last you can see what he looks like, and have your first embrace.

Your feelings may be a little overwhelming: intense relief that the birth is over may be followed by **a rush of love** as you cradle him. Or you may be shocked and exhausted after a grueling labor. It's quite likely you'll run through a whole gamut of emotions—euphoric one minute, then tearful and concerned the next as you wonder how you'll look after your tiny bundle. Don't worry if you're not instantly bowled over; **deep bonding** usually develops over the weeks and months. It's likely, though, that you'll feel instinctively protective of your baby and want to be near him.

You can prepare for how your baby might look: he'll emerge covered in blood and **vernix**—the white, waxy substance that coated his skin in the uterus—and he may be stained with **meconium**, the first tarry, black stool. If you had a vaginal birth, his head may be elongated from **squeezing through the birth canal,** his nose squashed, and eyes swollen. Rest assured that within a day or so all this settles down.

As soon as you can, hold your baby against you for **skin-to-skin contact**. This is very relaxing for both you and your baby, and research has shown that it helps to regulate your baby's **body temperature** and **stabilize his blood sugar levels**. He can hear the sound of your heartbeat, reminding him of being in the uterus. Holding him close to you helps prepare you both for breast-feeding and, in fact, increases the likelihood of successful breast-feeding; **such closeness also boosts his immunity**, because the bacteria on your skin transfers to your baby's skin. Skin-to-skin contact with Dad carries many of the same benefits, so dads should make sure they get in on all the cuddle action.

Did you know?

✳ Babies' cries reflect the "accent" of their mother tongue, suggesting that babies tune into their parents' language while in the uterus. Researchers found that French babies cried with a rising accent, while German babies had a falling inflection.

{ *It's often claimed that newborns resemble their dads, but studies reveal that this isn't always the case. One theory is that looking alike is an evolutionary device to ensure dads invest in the newborn. It's mothers who most often remark on the resemblance—perhaps a conditioned response to reassure dad that the baby is definitely his!* }

✳ Despite all that howling, newborns don't produce "real" tears. The undeveloped tear ducts produce just enough moisture to keep the eye healthy, but it will be several weeks before actual tears appear!

✳ If your baby has his own special birthmark, he's not alone. About 1 in 10 babies have some form of birthmark, the most common being port-wine stains and "stork" marks.

✳ Babies recognize their mothers from birth by smell and voice alone, showing a preference for their mother's breast milk and responding to her voice.

✳ A newborn's head is proportionally very large at one-quarter of his total body length. His brain accounts for around 10 percent of his total body weight. The rest of his body will now grow to catch up.

Your *baby* from top to toe

Before your newborn leaves the hospital, a staff pediatrician will give her a routine, hands-on examination.

This new baby top-to-toe checkup is designed to pick up anything untoward at the earliest opportunity. In addition to the checks below, your baby's pulse points and reflexes will be checked along with a careful visual examination of her skin, a count of her fingers and toes, and observation of her general well-being.

head In addition to measuring your baby's head circumference, the doctor will check your baby's soft spots, also known as his fontanelles.

eyes Babies' eyes are often puffy when they're newborns but that's normal. The doctor will want to assess their appearance and their position on the head. They'll also check her red reflex using an ophthalmoscope.

ears Ears come in all shapes and sizes and your baby's will be examined to see that they're sitting at about the right level and that they're intact and any skin tags are noted.

mouth To rule out certain physical defects, your doctor will look inside your baby's mouth and feel the roof of her mouth before going on to check her sucking reflex.

abdomen Your doctor will use firm pushes and prods to assess the size of your baby's internal organs.

heart & lungs

The doctor will want to listen to your baby's heart and lungs using a stethoscope to make sure that all is as it should be.

hips & back

Your baby's hips will be checked for any "clickiness" by bending them up and gently circling them. The bones of your baby's back are checked while she is face down.

feet The overall shape of your baby's feet and whether they're curled or twisted will be assessed. A tiny sample of blood from a heel prick will be taken (in the hospital) and tested for some rare but serious metabolic disorders.

genitals

These can be swollen in both baby girls and boys. They'll be checked to make sure everything looks and feels normal.

Hello *baby*

After the drama of labor and birth, you, your partner, and your new baby will have time alone to meet each other, reflect, and absorb the incredible newness of it all.

How you might feel

New moms may feel spaced out and somewhat euphoric over the coming day or so. Exhaustion from labor and birth combines with lingering pregnancy hormones and drugs, and those hormones released during feeding provide a natural high. Dads are likely to feel dazed, elated, and exhausted, too, and—of course—immensely proud. After an initial fairly alert period, your baby may spend much of his time sleeping, waking occasionally, and rooting to find your nipple. You may find he is more settled in your arms, needing the comfort of your closeness having spent nine months nestled in your uterus. This recuperative time offers the perfect chance simply to "be" with your baby and start to bond.

Mutual fascination

It's hard to take your eyes off your tiny new baby, so don't be surprised if you get nothing done but baby-gazing for a little while. Take your time to get to know him, taking in each feature, from his squashed nose to his

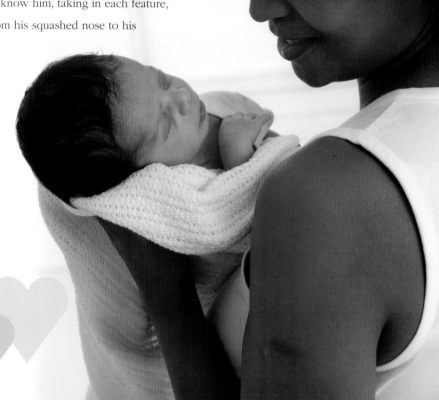

eyelashes, downy hair, and tiny fingernails. When he opens his eyes, your baby will fix on your face—this is the start of a mutual fascination that will grow into a loving bond.

Highs and lows

You may look back on these first days as ones of vivid and magnified emotions. The joy of being with your baby can overwhelm you one moment, while the next you're trying to figure out practical matters such as taking a shower. You may feel shocked at how alien your body feels as you grapple with feeding and dealing with post-birth discomfort. You may also feel strangely "empty." Rest assured all these emotional swings are completely normal.

Home or hospital

Your post-birth experience is influenced by your environment. Usually within an hour of a hospital birth, you will be transferred to the postpartum ward, which you'll share with other woman. The bustle and activity can make it hard to rest, and you may want to close your cubicle curtains for privacy. Private rooms are sometimes available. If you need to stay in for longer than usual, you'll also need to adjust to the routine of set mealtimes and hospital rounds. However, many women find a hospital environment deeply reassuring, with nurses available around the clock to offer help and advice, and other new parents providing camaraderie and mutual support. If you had a home birth, (which is very uncommon in the US), you should be able to relax and sleep more easily, which can help your recovery enormously. Just being able to sleep in your own bed and go into your own kitchen for a snack can help you settle into a daily routine.

> When your baby cries out, trust your instincts and do what feels right and natural.

REM sleep

Newborns spend 50 percent of their sleeping hours in light rapid eye movement (REM) sleep—more than double the time adults spend in this phase. This stage of sleep is a time of high brain activity, when the neural pathways associated with learning are stimulated. During REM, babies are quite restless and can wake up easily.

Getting a grip

One of the most daunting aspects of new parenthood is figuring out how to hold and handle your tiny new baby. Support his head and body and bring your body to his when you pick him up so he's not suspended in air. Be guided by his response—babies love to be held close, and if he looks comfortable then its unlikely that you're holding him too tightly.

For crying out loud!

Not only do you have a brand-new baby, but you're also about to learn a brand-new way of communicating. Your first day together introduces you to what will become a familiar sound—your baby's cry. Studies reveal that we are primed to respond with speed to a baby's cries, suggesting an evolved response that triggers us to help a baby in need. When your baby cries, you experience an urge to pick him up. This is more than just a simple reaction; your body actually has an ingrained, biological response to the sound of him crying, as the blood flow to your breasts increases and you feel a need to cradle him. When you are breast-feeding, release of the hormone oxytocin relaxes you and enhances your maternal response. Yet dads also feel this same protective instinct, toward their baby as well as toward their partner.

How to *soothe* your baby

Babies cry—that's a fact. Most young babies cry for between one and three hours a day since it's the only way they can communicate, but you will soon figure out what your baby is trying to tell you.

The most common reason for a baby to cry is that she is hungry or thirsty, but she could also be telling you that she feels tired, needs to be held, feels bored or lonely, is a little cold or hot, or just feels uncomfortable. A baby might also cry if her diaper needs changing and it feels wet against her skin. As you get to know your baby you will have a better sense of why she cries, and a pattern might emerge. If you already know your baby is clean, comfortable, and has been fed, it can be very useful to have some soothing strategies at hand. The key is to keep calm, and even if you don't figure out the cause, hopefully by the time she has settled back down you'll both be feeling better.

Declutter her mind

When your baby becomes overly tired she can find it difficult to fall asleep. Hold her facing a blank wall to block distractions, or hold a burp cloth in front of her carriage or car seat (don't let it cover her face).

Offer soothing words

Talk quietly to her, using a low, calm voice. "Shh…shh…shh" echoes the sounds she would have heard in the uterus. If she is lying down, stroke her in time with your soothing words. Singing and humming can work, too.

Sucking for comfort

A newborn's need to suck is strong and your breast or finger (or a pacifier) can offer comfort. This deep, comfort-sucking steadies your baby's heart rate and relaxes her stomach muscles.

Get moving

Gentle rocking can work wonders as its steady motion reminds her of being in the uterus. Try walking around as you rock her, sit together in a rocking chair, or rock her in a gentle bouncy chair. The motion of being in the carriage, front carrier, or car can calm a baby and send her to sleep. Going for a walk can benefit both of you since the motion of walking, the swaying trees, the sights and sounds of a park, or low traffic noise can be very soothing to baby and parents!

Hold her close

Your baby is soothed by you, so start by picking her up and holding her close to you. She will feel your heartbeat, warmth, and strong, comforting presence. Gently rub her back or tummy in a soft, rhythmic motion. Carrying her in a front pack, or lying with her skin-to-skin can also be very calming. Putting your baby down in her bassinet or crib could be the answer, too, especially if she is tired or overstimulated from lots of holding and attention.

Rhythmic relaxation

In the uterus your baby could hear the beat of your heart and the gurgle of your stomach, and being held close to you reminds her of that. Other repetitive noises have a similar calming effect such as the "white noise" of a dishwasher, vacuum, or hair dryer. You can download apps or buy CDs compiled specifically for babies that contain soothing music and natural sounds such as the sea.

Stroke and caress her

Stroke her head, back, and face gently as you hold her close. Baby massage (see pages 148–149) can be a useful technique, particularly with a colicky baby or if your baby is fussy before bedtime.

Often, all your baby needs is your comforting presence and the deep reassurance she finds in your touch. Knowing you are there soothes her cries and enables her to let go and relax in the security of your love.

Super survival instincts

Unable to control her movements or choose a safe environment, how does your newborn baby cope in the outside world? Enter Mom and Dad…

Your baby is born with an **amazing set of skills** to help her survive, and to encourage you to take care of her. Those big eyes, cute hands, and determined cry prove very useful in making parents do all the hard work. Your baby is also born with a set of **primitive reflexes** that provide clues to our evolutionary past, and although they vary in usefulness today, some are still crucial for survival.

Babies are born with about 70 primitive reflexes. The most familiar include the essential **rooting and sucking reflexes** that she needs to find food. As you stroke your baby's cheek, she'll turn and root for food, whether the breast or bottle, then suck automatically. The **protective Moro (or startle) reflex** occurs when your baby is startled by a noise or movement: she throws back her head, flings out her arms, then pulls them back to her body. Particularly endearing is the **grasp reflex**: if you place your finger in your baby's palm, she will grip it strongly and won't let go! This continues with gripping your hair and clothes. When you support your baby upright, with her feet on a flat surface, her legs will work with a **stepping reflex**. Babies can't walk at this age, but she may be born with an innate knowledge of how to walk that will be put into practice when her body is stronger.

Healthy newborn reflexes indicate that your baby's **nervous system is functioning as it should**, and they will be checked by your doctor when your baby is born. In the following weeks and months, newborn reflexes fade and your baby will figure out how to control his movements, and before you know it he will be helping himself to cookies and whizzing around exploring the world.

Did you know?

✳ **Newborns placed under water can
hold their breath and move their limbs in a swimming motion.
Don't try this at home! These diving and swimming reflexes are for
survival only and don't mean your baby can swim.**

*Some reflexes have more than one use: grasping was
important when mammals had to cling to their mother's
fur, but it also promotes bonding, helping the parents feel
loved. Sucking, which is essential for baby's survival, is
also a primary source of his comfort.*

✳ Babies may be
designed to breast-feed lying down.
A 2008 study observed that newborns use
17 reflexes to nurse when their mother lies
down, compared with just three when fed
upright. The same moms reported greater
success breast-feeding when
lying down.

✳ Children are born to be active,
to wiggle, wave arms, and run around.
Experts have found evidence that older
children who still demonstrate their
primitive reflexes may benefit from
more physical exercise, and may have
spent too much time sitting still
in a stroller.

✳ **Primitive reflexes, especially the rooting, grasp, and startle ones,
indicate that babies are "passive parent clingers," meaning they are
designed to want to be held close. In the 1970s, Colombian
research established "kangaroo" care for premature
babies, finding that babies thrived when held
close with skin-to-skin contact.**

Sleeping like a *baby*

The subject of babies' sleep is laden with conflicting advice and opinions. So just how do you decide who to listen to?

Deciding where and how you put your baby to sleep can seem like a terrifyingly trap-laden prospect. You'll read rules about night wear and room temperature, type of mattress and covers. Many such recommendations stem from research into sudden infant death syndrome and in certain countries health professionals can only advocate conditions that are borne of such studies. Whether you follow the prescribed route or make your own way in the sleeping scene is up to you.

Our parents and grandparents had different practices, just like parents around the world today. Take your baby's first bed. Do you opt for a Moses basket, a crib, or bassinet? And should it be attached to your mattress, within arm's reach, on the bed, or in another room? The right answer depends on where you live. Side-by-side futons are popular in Japan. In Central and South America and in the Pacific, **babies sleep in hammocks**: the cocoon of fabric feels comforting, allows air to circulate, and keeps the baby safely facing upward; and as she shifts in her sleep, the baby sets up a rocking motion that lulls her through periods of waking. Some neonatal intensive care units (NICUs) have even adapted hammocks for these reasons. **Swaddling babies** for sleep is routine practice across former Soviet countries, South America, and the Middle East, whereas **strapping babies to cradleboards** is common among Native Americans for its similarly soothing effects.

Does your baby share your bed? Join the gang. A study found that up to 71 percent of parents and babies across the globe sleep body-to-body. Some, though, consider this a bridge too far, since retiring to your own bed is one of the few opportunities parents get to have a moment of privacy. Furthermore co-sleeping comes with cautions—bedding might smother or overheat the baby, a tipsy mom or dad could roll on top of her, or she might get wedged between bed and wall. But in many countries, including Japan

Proponents of co-sleeping believe that it helps babies feel secure, in turn promoting confidence and independence as they grow.

and China, **co-sleeping is normal practice**, and it continues until babies are big wiggly children, even teenagers. In fact, it is considered bad parenting to not sleep with a child, or to expect privacy in bed. The Japanese refer to it as river-sleeping—the parents forming the safe banks with the baby shifting between.

Advocates of co-sleeping have produced data showing that in countries where this is the norm, the **rate of sudden infant death syndrome is among the lowest in the industrialized world**, possibly because sleeping together is thought to help babies regulate their temperature better, and that the sound of an adult's breathing and movement of a mother's chest encourage similar healthy patterns in infants.

However, don't worry—or feel guilty!—if you fall into the large category of parents who simply can't countenance the idea of sharing a bed with their baby each night. For many parents, moving a baby into **a crib in a separate room** is a milestone that represents the beginning of a return to autonomy. With their baby safely in the nursery, parents can extend bedtime (co-sleeping means never leaving an infant alone in bed), there's no need to be entirely sober, and adult activities can return to the parental bed—even if reading with the light on beats the thought of sex. Many modern parents like to be **independent of their children at night**, believing it promotes independence, and that by coddling babies they will become clingy and unable to manage alone.

How often your society expects a baby to rest, nap, and be stimulated can affect sleep patterns. The American expectation that babies need to be active, learn, and spend time away from parents means they get less sleep than babies in China, where **rest and quietness**, protection, and dependence have more emphasis; or in the Netherlands, where an **early bedtime is sacrosanct**. Bedtime routines are cultural, too. Mayan parents in Guatemala let children fall asleep whenever and wherever; US and UK families tend to have **set bedtime rituals** to herald a parent leaving.

Perhaps the most tricky expectation is for babies to **sleep through the night**—something almost all new parents crave. Researchers say it is biologically inappropriate: until their first birthday babies wake for food and "socio-emotional" reasons. They are hardwired for sensory communication— tactile, visual, auditory, olfactory—even at night.

Though it's possible, through sleep training, to encourage your baby not to bother you at night, try to remember that, to an extent, **night waking is simply a part of being human**. Babies are not ready to operate independently at birth, and since separation from the caregiver is one of the surest life-threatening situations, it's no wonder the infant brain and nervous system is primed to protest.

Early parenthood is a time of adaptation: accepting inevitable sleep disruptions removes much of the associated anxiety.

If you are stressed about your baby not sleeping, many experienced mothers would say ignore the mind-boggling sleep charts and programs, and **just do what feels right for you and your baby**—whether that involves a bout of controlled crying or bringing your baby into bed. As long as you are satisfied that she is safe, dry, full, and healthy, you are not going to introduce any long-term negative effects through your choice of sleeping method.

Simply the breast

From the moment your baby is born, your body continues to provide nourishment, switching its focus from feeding him via the placenta to establishing a milk supply through your breasts. Milk production is underway and your breasts are gearing up for the job at hand.

It takes a few days for your breast milk to come in, but there's a good reason to start nursing right away, since your breasts are primed to deliver the "pre-milk" colostrum, the production of which started in mid-pregnancy. Dubbed "liquid gold" for its remarkable composition, colostrum is a golden yellow and produced in tiny quantities. Your baby receives just a few teaspoons' worth in the first days, perfectly suited to his tiny stomach (which is the size of a walnut).

A liquid gold mine
Rich in nutrients, colostrum contains three times as much protein (including all the essential aminio acids) as mature milk, and is coated in fat-soluble vitamins and minerals. It's low in carbohydrate, fat, and lactose, and high in sodium, potassium, and cholesterol, which assist growth of the brain, heart, and nervous system. Colostrum also acts as a laxative, stimulating the passage of meconium, and in doing so reduces your baby's risk of jaundice.

Time for milk

Frequent sucking in the first days stimulates milk production, and on days three to five your milk "comes in." This first milk—"transitional" milk—has less protein and fewer antibodies, but is high in fat, calories, and lactose to meet your growing baby's needs. It's what he'll enjoy for the next week or so before "mature" milk arrives. The quantity is far greater so you may find your breasts suddenly uncomfortably full. Letting your baby nurse eases the pressure, and production will even out.

A two-course meal

During each breast-feeding the makeup of your milk changes. The first milk—foremilk—is a watery mixture to quench your baby's thirst. Once the ledown reflex is triggered by this early feeding, the hindmilk is released; this rich milk supplies energy and body-building proteins for growth and development and fills him up.

Immune boosters

In addition to antibodies, breast milk contains lactoferrin (which combats infection), lysozyme (which enhances antibody activity), mucins (which stick to microbes to get rid of them), and white blood cells (which actively fight germs). So, breast-feeding is one of the best ways to boost your baby's health.

A changeable feast

COLOSTRUM									BIRTH	COLOSTRUM					TRANSITIONAL MILK				
9	8	7	6	5	4	3	2	1		1	2	3	4	5	6	7	8	9	10

days before birth | days after birth

Your breasts start to produce colostrum some time in your second trimester.

Colostrum is packed with white blood cells and antibodies

The volume and nature of milk changes over the next ten days.

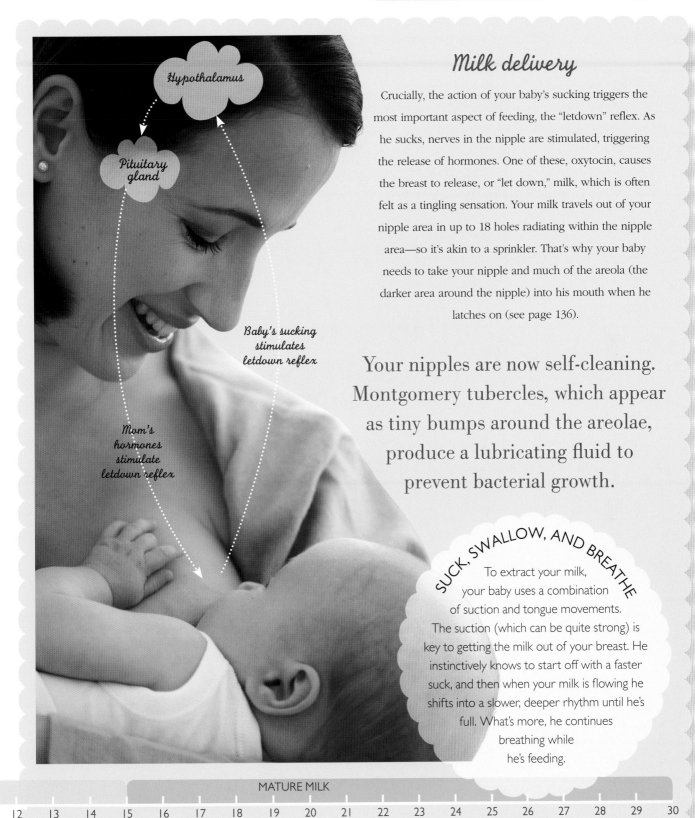

Hypothalamus

Pituitary gland

Baby's sucking stimulates letdown reflex

Mom's hormones stimulate letdown reflex

Milk delivery

Crucially, the action of your baby's sucking triggers the most important aspect of feeding, the "letdown" reflex. As he sucks, nerves in the nipple are stimulated, triggering the release of hormones. One of these, oxytocin, causes the breast to release, or "let down," milk, which is often felt as a tingling sensation. Your milk travels out of your nipple area in up to 18 holes radiating within the nipple area—so it's akin to a sprinkler. That's why your baby needs to take your nipple and much of the areola (the darker area around the nipple) into his mouth when he latches on (see page 136).

Your nipples are now self-cleaning. Montgomery tubercles, which appear as tiny bumps around the areolae, produce a lubricating fluid to prevent bacterial growth.

SUCK, SWALLOW, AND BREATHE

To extract your milk, your baby uses a combination of suction and tongue movements. The suction (which can be quite strong) is key to getting the milk out of your breast. He instinctively knows to start off with a faster suck, and then when your milk is flowing he shifts into a slower, deeper rhythm until he's full. What's more, he continues breathing while he's feeding.

MATURE MILK

| 12 | 13 | 14 | 15 | 16 | 17 | 18 | 19 | 20 | 21 | 22 | 23 | 24 | 25 | 26 | 27 | 28 | 29 | 30 |

days after birth

Your milk will reflect what you eat, so will taste different each day.

Top *feeding* positions

Once you get the hang of breast-feeding, you can feed your baby anywhere and any way you feel comfortable. In the early weeks, you may breast-feed for up to an hour at a time, so you will need to find a position (there are several) that allows you to relax and that won't leave your arms, neck, or back feeling sore.

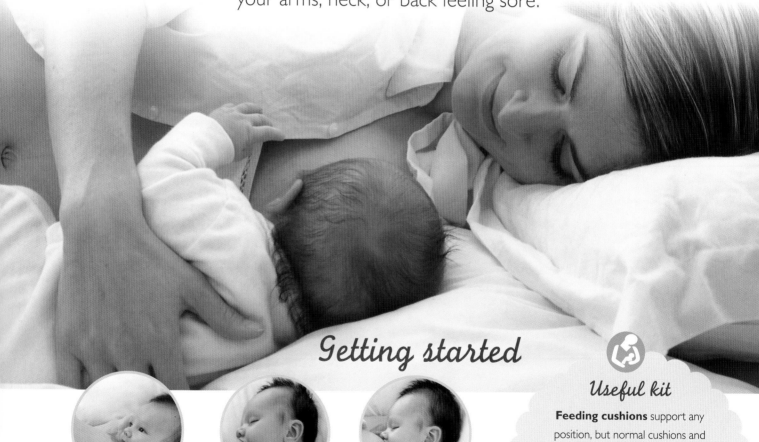

Getting started

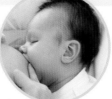

Useful kit

Feeding cushions support any position, but normal cushions and pillows are fine, too. **Burp cloths** mop up milk and cover your baby's head, preserving modesty, and keeping baby's attention focused. **Lanolin-based nipple creams** can be a godsend in the early weeks to moisturize, soothe, and protect sore nipples.

Get in place
Brushing your nipple against your baby's lip prompts his mouth to open ready for the nipple.

Latching on
When it is wide open, quickly bring his mouth to your nipple, taking in as much areola as possible.

And…release
Slip a finger into his mouth to break the suction, then quickly move his head away from your breast.

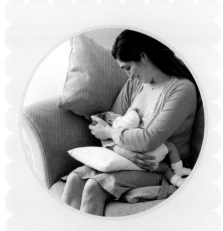

Cradle hold

You are likely to use this hold most often, especially if you breast-feed in public. Get comfortable on a chair with a cushion behind your lower back so you are straight and supported. Lift your baby up and onto your breast so she lies across your body, facing you, with her body in a straight line. Support her head in the fold of your arm. When she is tiny, you might need pillows to raise her level with your breast.

Football hold

An under-the-arm position is good when in bed or on the sofa, when you have pillows or cushions to place at your side. Tuck baby under your arm, with her legs and body wrapped around your side and resting on the cushions. Bring her to your breast, supporting her head and neck. This position is ideal after a cesarean since there is no weight on your abdomen.

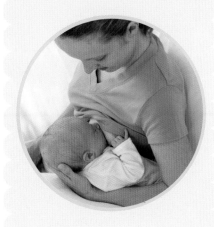

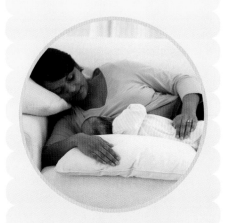

Reclining hold

Lying next to your baby can be a lovely way to breast-feed, especially at night because you can stay in bed! Bring her to your breast (perhaps resting on a pillow so she is at the right height), with your tummies close together, and support her with your arm so she can't roll away. When you want to change breasts, you will need to roll over to your other side, so carefully move your baby then reposition.

Toughening up

Breast-feeding takes practice, so don't be disheartened if it doesn't work right away. Until your nipples toughen up they will be sensitive, but if feeding is excessively painful your baby may not be latched on correctly. Talk to your doctor about breast-feeding support groups.

Out and about

Playgroups and baby classes are all places where mothers regularly breast-feed, so there is no need to worry or feel self-conscious about breast-feeding in public. Using a cradle hold makes this particularly easy. A long cardigan, wrap, or nursing top can help give you a little extra privacy, and you could practice in front of a mirror to check what others can (or can't) see.

DID YOU KNOW?

In the UK between 2005 and 2010, the percentage of newborns who were (initially) breast-fed rose from 78 percent to 83 percent.

Using different feeding positions helps you to empty your breasts completely of milk.

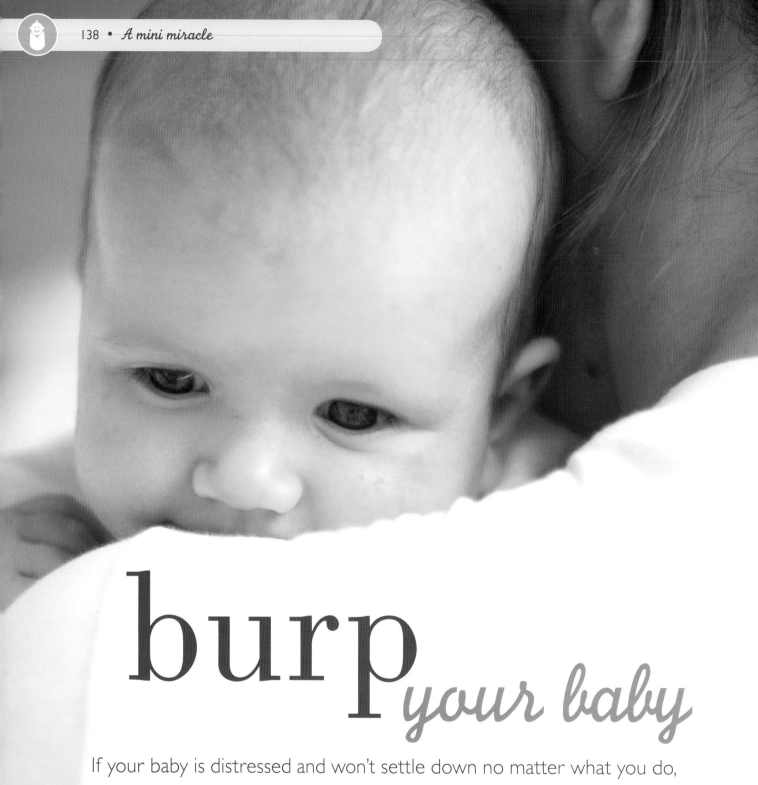

burp *your baby*

If your baby is distressed and won't settle down no matter what you do, the problem could be trapped gas. There are various positions you can try to release the air, and different babies respond to different techniques. Experiment with these positions to see what works best for your baby.

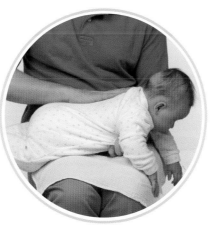

Lying across the lap
This position allows your baby's weight to press on his tummy. Hold under his arms and rub his back to displace any trapped gas.

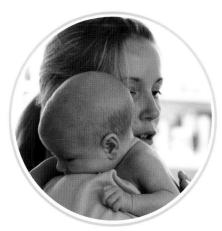

Up and over the shoulder
Position him so his tummy, not his chest, rests against your shoulder and pat his back to release any trapped gas. This soothing and comfortable position, allows you to walk around while burping him.

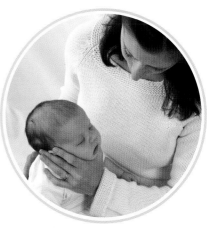

Sitting with the chin up
Straightening up his body can help bring up a burp or two. Bring him up to a sitting position, then slowly lean him forward while supporting and raising his chin. Firmly rub his back in a circular motion.

> It doesn't matter from which end the gas exits your baby, just as long as it comes out eventually.

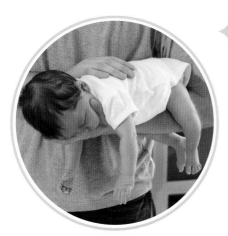

Lying along the arm
Babies enjoy the new view of the world this position offers. Tuck him into the crook of your elbow with his tummy along your hand or arm and rub his back. Walking can also help jiggle out the gas.

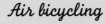

Air bicycling
This is a fun way of releasing gas and relieving tummy aches. Stretch out one of his legs while pushing the other one so it bends in close to his body. Alternate each side to emulate a cycling movement.

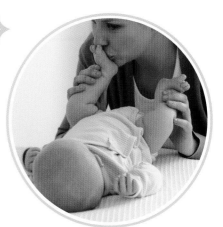

Toes meet nose
Similar to air bicycling, moving your baby's toes up to his nose can ease crampy gas pains. Lie him on the floor or on your lap and push his legs forward until his toes touch his nose. It's effective and seems like fun at the same time.

Beautiful
bottlefeeding

Most babies will be fed using a bottle at some point, either right from the start, when starting solids, or when Mom has to return to work. So, step up, Daddy, it's feeding time!

Successfully teaching your baby to take a bottle can be hugely beneficial for you, your baby, and your partner. If you are formula-feeding then your baby will acquire this skill from day one, but if you breast-feed it can be more of a challenge. Feeding your baby is a wonderfully bonding experience, and one of the key advantages of bottle-feeding is that it offers a great opportunity for your partner—as well as others, such as doting grandparents, aunts, or friends—to share in such moments. It can be liberating to think that feeding baby is not your sole responsibilty, day and night—and it means that you will be able to indulge in the occasional night out! Bottle-feeding means your baby doubles up on his parental bonding, and your life can be a bit more flexible.

From breast to bottle

Once breast-feeding is well established—usually from about six weeks—you could try expressing milk. Getting your baby to accept a bottle can take some persuasion, so initially she might be happier taking a bottle from someone else, since she will associate you with feeding and will be able to smell your breast milk, which may upset her.

Express yourself

Expressing milk is easy, painless, and relatively quick. A hand pump is probably all you need if you only plan to express every once in a while, but if you need a regular supply, for instance if you are returning to work or storing it to go away, it might be a good idea to invest in an electric pump since they are faster and more efficient.

The ideal time to express is in the morning after your baby has had a full feeding since your milk will be richest and most plentiful at this time. Breasts are self-regulating, so if you get into the habit of expressing after your baby is done feeding, your body will learn to produce extra milk at this time of day.

Getting comfortable

Your baby loves being held close to you as you nurse him. Make sure your back is straight and bring your baby up to your chest height so he can gaze into your eyes: use a cushion under him for support so you are not bending over. Talk to your baby as you feed him and let him pause if he needs a break or to burp him. Change sides to give your arm a rest.

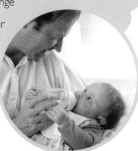

Milk etiquette

Expressed breast milk needs to be stored in the refrigerator (or freezer, see below) so it doesn't go bad. You can keep fresh breast milk in the refrigerator for 72 hours, in bottles or designated bags. If your baby doesn't finish a feeding, you will need to throw the rest of the milk away. Formula should be made up fresh each time, although opened, ready-to-use cartons can be refrigerated for up to 48 hours. Milk can be served warm, cold, or at room temperature.

Freezing milk
Breast milk can be refrigerated for three to eight days or frozen for 6 to 12 months; you can buy sterile, sealable bags. It is not safe to freeze formula.

Sterilizing
Pumps, bottles, and nipples all need to be cleaned thoroughly but it's not necessary to sterilize equipment repeatedly, after the initial sterilization (following the manufacturer's instructions, which often involves boiling in water for ten minutes). It's fine to wash the parts in your dishwasher after that.

Making up the formula

1. Boil the water, then allow it to cool for about half an hour.

2. Measure the cooled boiled water into a clean bottle.

3. Add the right number of level spoonfuls of formula powder.

4. Secure the lid and shake to dissolve it all.

5. Before feeding your baby, test the temperature on your skin.

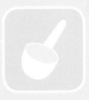

Measuring
Accuracy is vital with formula: if it is too strong a baby can become dehydrated; if it is too weak she will be hungry. Most formulas allow 1 oz (30 ml) water per scoop of powder. As a rough guide, each day a baby should drink 5–7 floz (150–200 ml) formula per 2 lb (1 kg) of body weight.

Body-boosting foods
for mom

As a new mom, you need all the energy you can get. Don't rush into losing the pregnancy pounds; instead eat energy-boosting, nutrient-rich foods at regular intervals to help your post-birth body recover quickly.

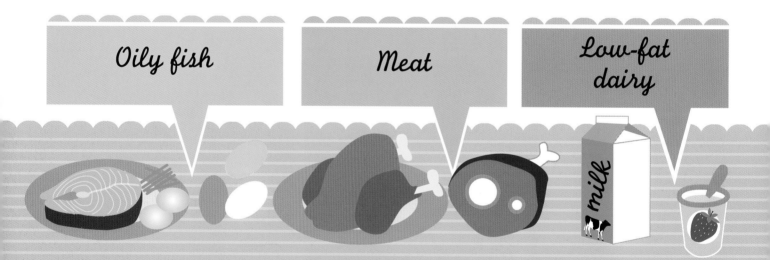

Oily fish

Meat

Low-fat dairy

Oily fish, such as salmon, herring, sardines, and mackerel, are loaded with a fatty acid (docosahexaenoic acid, or **DHA** for short), which is essential for normal brain function and a healthy heart. Studies show it may also help **prevent postpartum depression** and **elevate your mood.** Limit it to 12 oz (340 g) a week to prevent overexposure to mercury. Omega-3 fortified eggs are another source of DHA.

A deficiency of iron, which can happen after birth-related blood loss, can drain your energy levels. Lean beef is **high in iron,** which can help replenish your supply. Also, all meat contains **body-repairing proteins** (and vegetarian proteins do too), so include these in snacks or main meals to recharge your body after the work of labor.

If you are breast-feeding, your milk stays pretty much the same quality no matter what you eat, because your body prioritizes nutrients for your baby and can take from your body whatever's missing from your diet. Eating plenty of **calcium-rich foods,** such as **yogurt, milk, and cheese** (as well as green leafy vegetables) ensures your own bones stay strong.

You are two-thirds water

Try to drink about 2 pints (1.2 liters) of fluids a day.

Other fluids

No need to limit yourself to water; milk and fruit juices also count.

Dehydration is one of the biggest drains on your energy levels, so be on top of your fluid intake. If you're not normally a water drinker, pop in a slice of lemon or lime to add extra flavor. And you'll get about 1¾ pints (1 liter) of water from your food.

It feels counterintuitive, but drinking plenty of water helps to prevent fluid retention.

Whole-grain cereal

Fruit and vegetables

Dark chocolate

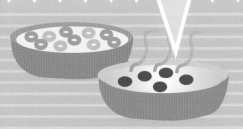

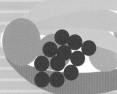

choc

If you're struggling with the little amount of restorative sleep that comes with taking care of a newborn, then you need a **morning power shot** to start your day. Whole-grain cereals **boost energy,** and many are fortified with essential vitamins and nutrients. For cold days, try some warming **oatmeal** topped with a handful of antioxidant-rich blueberries.

Grab a piece of **fruit** for a quick pick-me-up to give you energy without the "crash" of junk food, and for a **fiber boost,** which keeps your digestive tract moving. **Leafy greens,** including spinach, Swiss chard, and broccoli, are packed with **vitamins (A and C), iron, and a nondairy source of calcium,** so they're perfect postpartum ingredients.

High-quality dark chocolate—with cocoa levels of **70 percent or higher**—is a treat that comes with benefits. It can improve your mood by **increasing serotonin** levels in the brain; some studies show it might trigger the release of **endorphins,** the body's feel-good chemicals. But, chocolate does contain caffeine, so choose wisely the time of day to indulge.

Dads do it like this...

Roll up your sleeves and get ready to join the club of 21st-century fathers, who take an active role in raising a baby.

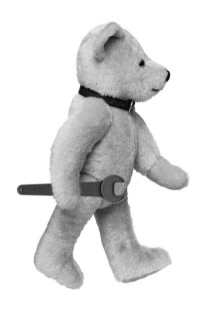

Dads who actively bond with their babies from day one not only boost their child's physical and mental development, but also hold the key to their family's strength as a unit, and even to their child's future attitudes and their likelihood of success in life. Children whose fathers bonded with them at an early age tend to be academically more successful, emotionally more secure, use drugs and alcohol less frequently, and are less likely to get involved with crime. No pressure there! It seems we've come a long way from the days when a father was expected to stay firmly in the role of **protector, breadwinner, and disciplinarian** and rarely had much involvement in their child's early upbringing at all.

A baby's brain development and emotional stability relates directly to a father's involvement during the early years of life.

But is it all just about dividing up the chores, sharing the yucky jobs, and helping with the practical demands of having a new baby? On the contrary, experts say that what new dads are really needed for is bonding. Good, old-fashioned, **gooey-at-the-knees bonding**. This is great news for many dads, who are enthusiastic at getting in on the cuddling action. But it can be a challenge for those who are unsure where to begin—and whose own fathers may not have bonded well with them, limited as they were by a different generation's expectations. So, how can you bond—and what's in it for you?

Experts stress that you shouldn't feel you have to be a kind of "second mom." You're a dad, do it your way—that's what your baby needs. Often moms are more organized, for instance remembering snacks when going out, and anticipating the need for sleep, comforters, and entertainment. Dads tend to be more relaxed and are far more likely to "wing it" under the mantra that if you don't have it, you can always buy it. Men play more **"rough and tumble"** with their children, and encourage more risk-taking behavior. They also use a **different vocabulary**, often using complicated words (where mothers adjust their language down) that help to broaden the child's vocabulary. Yet these different methods of child care are complementary rather than antagonistic, since babies benefit from the two parenting styles—think of it as a mom's yin to dad's yang.

Fathers who familiarize themselves with their babies and attune to their needs, will increase their own confidence with their baby.

Bonding can be simple—a midnight feeding, a shared bath, hiding under a blanket to get a giggle. You could "wear" your baby in a baby carrier or sling, or read, sing, and listen to music together. If you really want to find a special bond you could do a new activity together, for example, baby swimming or **baby sign language**. Babies use their hands to express needs and feelings—if you can understand that language, and use it too, you'll grow closer.

Researchers in Canada and Israel have found that men experience a surge in "bonding" hormones when their children are born. Even during their wives' pregnancies, men display a shift in their levels of the stress hormone cortisol, as well as prolactin, a hormone linked to parenting behavior. At the same time, they experience a rise in oxytocin, a brain chemical that can **dilute a man's alpha-male attitude** and engender a more nurturing nature. It's an evolutionary response intended to turn "guys" into dads.

Despite all this, some fathers feel truly daunted by the financial and emotional responsibilities of parenthood. Traditionally **postpartum depression** is a condition associated with new mothers, but experts believe as many as one in four new dads may suffer from it. So, if you, as a dad, find yourself experiencing mood swings, panic attacks, or tearfulness, be reassured that it is not uncommon, but it is important to speak out—to your partner, your doctor, even your boss, or a trusted friend. **Dads need as much support** as moms, and you need time to rest too.

Perhaps you can take some inspiration from other dads across the world. Swedish fathers are apparently Europe's most "involved" dads, partly because they have more **paternity leave** than any other country. But in all Northern European countries, dads tend to get more involved since they don't have **big extended families** like those in Southern European countries, such as Greece, where grandmothers, sisters, and aunts help with a lot of the child care.

Across the globe, though, there has been a dramatic increase in the level of paternal involvement over the last few decades. Between 1965 and 2000 in the US, married fathers **more than doubled their time** spent exclusively on child-care activities, from 2.6 hours a week to 6.5 hours. Australian fathers' care of children has also risen, and in the UK, fathers in two-parent families today do an average of 25 percent of the child-care-related activities during the week and 30 percent on weekends.

For true inspiration, though, look to the Aka Pygmies, a nomadic people of the African Congo. The men in these communities, on average, hold, or are in close proximity to, their infants 47 percent of the time. They **pick up, cuddle, and play** with their babies at least five times as often as dads in other societies. They must know they're onto a good thing, so roll up your sleeves, get bonding, and enjoy becoming a father.

Baby *sense*-sational

Your baby has arrived into an amazing world and all she wants to do is to explore it. Her sensory organs began developing way back in the sixth week of pregnancy, so now she is ready to learn.

Hearing is believing

Sudden noises may startle your baby and, in contrast, she may be soothed by constant hums. Familiar voices she has heard in the uterus are also calming, because she has already learned that you provide food and comfort. At birth, babies cannot coordinate sight and sound, so will not look in the direction of a sound. Exposing her to music will fine tune her hearing.

Touchy feely

During her first three months, your baby will be exploring the different textures of the world for the first time. She will look to you for the soft touch, to show her how love, comfort, and reassurance can be provided through touch. Studies have shown that babies who are massaged develop quicker, and babies who are lovingly touched get sick less frequently, smile more, and don't cry as much. As if you needed any excuse for more cuddling.

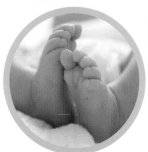

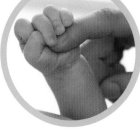

Taste sensation

Of course your baby will only be drinking milk, and she is programmed to enjoy its sweet taste. Later, once she starts to eat, she may be more adventurous if she has been breast-fed, since she will have grown accustomed to the way the taste of breast milk changes with your diet.

Scents of you

Your baby will instinctively turn away from unpleasant smells and toward nice ones. She will recognize your natural aroma and the fragrance of your beauty products; she will know it is you holding her even if she can't see you.

The light fantastic

A newborn's eyes are sensitive to light, so she is most likely to open her eyes in a darkened room. She is very nearsighted at birth and sees best at a distance of 8–12 in (20–30 cm), perfect for watching your face while she is feeding. Her eyes won't work together at first, so she may see two of everything, and her ability to perceive color will develop over her first four months. In addition to faces, she will most enjoy looking at strongly contrasting colors.

A one-week-old baby's sense of smell is so acute that she can distinguish her mother's breast milk from someone else's.

Your baby's senses

Hearing

This sense develops in the uterus but, once born, a baby still can't detect individual tones if there is a lot of background noise. This auditory function does not mature until a baby is five to six months old.

Touch

Babies use touch to explore their immediate environment. Their most sensitive touch receptors are in and around their mouths.

Motion

Newborns are used to the movement of your body from being in the uterus, so she will be soothed by a rocking motion.

Pressure and temperature

Receptors in her skin can sense types of pressure, heat, and cold. She may sense temperature but she can't yet tell you if she's too hot.

Newborn range of vision: 8–12 in (20–30 cm)

Sight

Your newborn's weak and unfocused eye muscles will strengthen within a matter of weeks. By three months she is able to watch her own hands while she uses them. This crucial step allows her to discover the amazing dexterity of her own hands, and helps her to develop hand–eye coordination.

Taste and smell

Babies are born with fully developed taste buds—these come with an built-in preference for sweet tastes and an aversion to anything bitter. As she grows, her taste preferences will adapt.

DID YOU KNOW?

In addition to their five main senses, all babies are born with the ability to detect a huge range of sensations, including heat, pain, gravity, and motion. Primitive eyes, ears, and limbs are visible after just six weeks of pregnancy.

In the mouth

In the coming months your baby will put everything in her mouth—to fully explore texture, shape, and taste.

The power of *touch*

Whether you choose to take your baby to special baby massage classes or opt for a do-it-yourself approach at home, what will become clear is the soothing power of this hands-on approach for your baby and you.

You might want to wait until your baby is six weeks old or so, when you find you have the time and energy to enjoy giving your baby a simple massage and then build this into your daily routine. The quiet time together, with plenty of smiles and eye contact is a wonderfully bonding one.

Massaging your baby has real health benefits: it reduces stress hormones, eases the symptoms of colds, colic, and teething, improves your baby's muscle tone, and stimulates growth hormones. And parents benefit, too: giving a massage can help to relax you and research has shown that it can alleviate postpartum depression.

The best times to get hands on are after your baby's bath time or in the morning when he is refreshed. Lay your baby on a towel in a warm room and use a baby massage oil or organic sunflower oil so your hands glide over his skin.

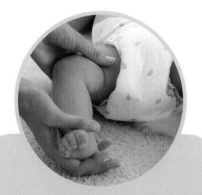

His legs

1

His legs are less sensitive than his hands and torso, and so make the best place to start since it won't startle him. Use a little oil, warmed in your hands, then wrap your hands around one thigh and pull gently down, one hand after the other, as if you are "milking" him. Squeeze gently as you go. Repeat with the other leg.

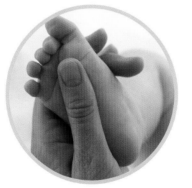

His feet

2

Move on to the first foot, and gently rotate it a few times in each direction. Stroke the top of his foot, from ankle to toes. Do the same with the other foot. Use your thumbs to trace small circles over the soles of each foot firmly, without tickling. To finish, take each toe between your thumb and forefinger and gently pull until the toe slips out of your fingers.

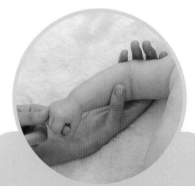

His arms

3

Do the same gentle motion you used on his legs on his arms. Start at each armpit and go down to each wrist. Take each hand and gently rotate his wrist a few times in each direction. Go on to trace circles with your thumbs on the palm of each hand. To finish, take each finger between your thumb and forefinger and pull gently until they slip through.

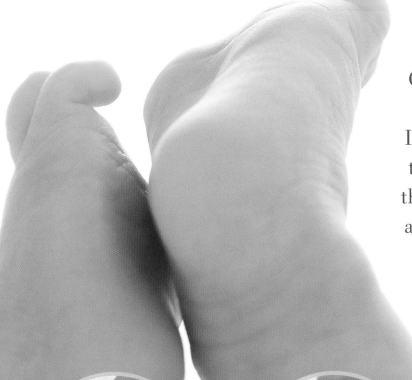

Gentle massage can help alleviate trapped gas. If your baby suffers from this, add an extra step to the sequence (after step 4) and stroke his belly using clockwise motions.

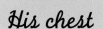

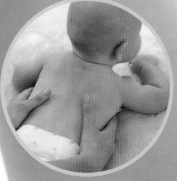

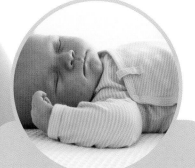

His chest

Place your hands together palms down on the center of his chest and stroke outward in large circles. Repeat these moves a few times. Place one hand flat on his chest and stroke it down to his thighs then repeat using alternate hands in a rhythmic movement.

His back

Roll your baby gently on to his tummy. Use your fingertips to trace small circles down his spine. Then switch to longer strokes (as you used on his chest) from his shoulders down the length of his back to his feet, working in a regular rhythm.

Ahh... that's nice

Turn him over now and cuddle him. He may be ready for a feeding and then bed or if it's during the day a recuperative nap. The end result, whatever the time of day, is a content and relaxed baby.

Go to sleep, *my baby...*

A lullaby works its magic on your baby's brain with its simple rhythm and slow tempo, which is easy for her hearing system to deal with.

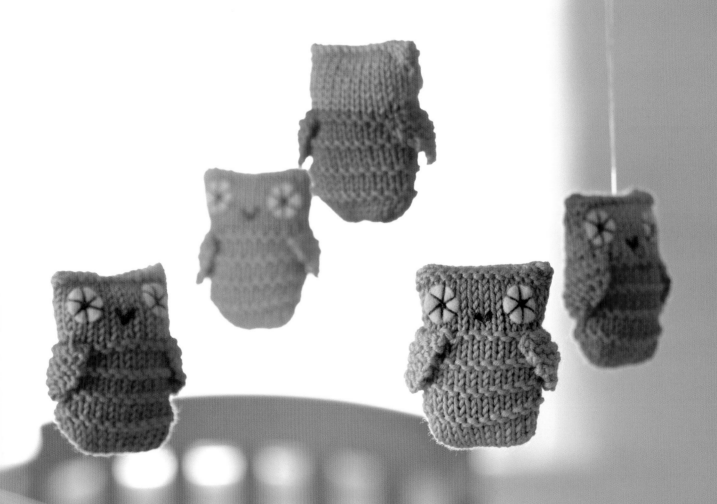

In the first week of life, babies sleep for a maximum of four hours at a time. But by the time they reach four months this has rocketed to over eight hours.

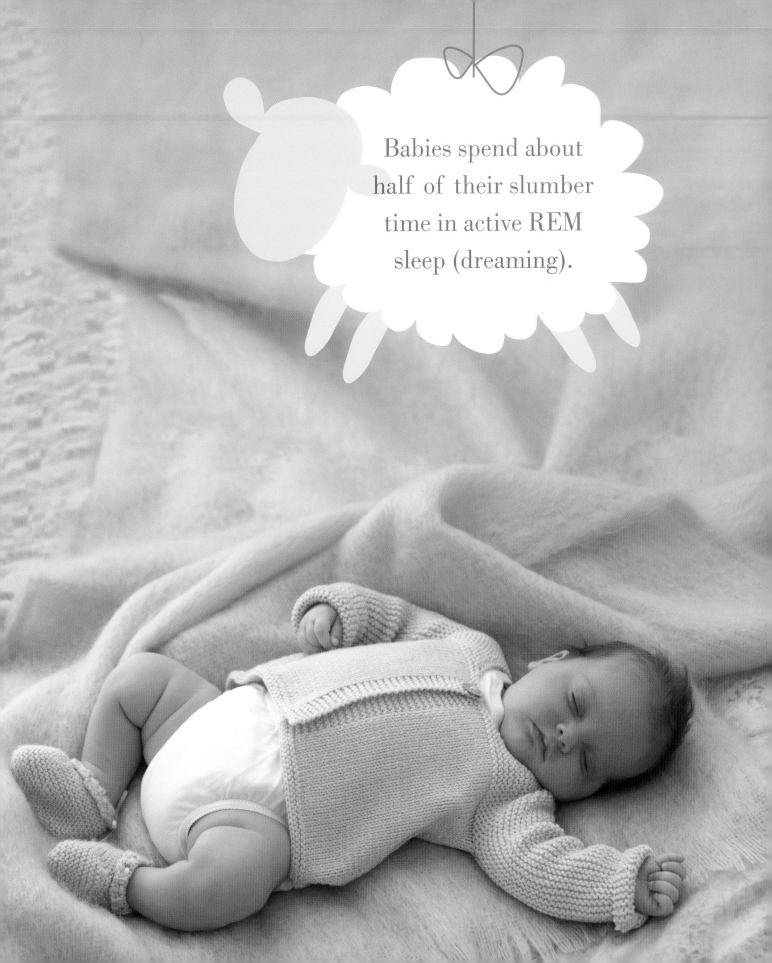

Babies spend about half of their slumber time in active REM sleep (dreaming).

Baby's bath-time

You've mastered feeding your baby, holding her, and changing her diaper, but then comes the anticipation of her first bath. Don't panic! In no time, you'll be looking forward to this chance to wind down with your baby.

Taking the plunge

Don't jump in! Before immersing your naked baby into water and holding her securely while you clean her you need to be well prepared. Gather a towel, a clean diaper and onesie, and anything else you need before you start so that you can give her your undivided attention. And stay calm—even if she protests, she'll learn from your relaxed approach that this is a perfectly normal turn of events.

Warm, but not too hot!

The temperature of the water is something you need to get just right. You don't want her shivering in water that's on the cold side, and you should definitely avoid immersing her in too-hot water. Aim for comfortably warm, using the front of your wrist (or elbow) to gauge the temperature or, to be extra sure, a bath thermometer (reading 100° F/38° C). A warm, draft-free room will add to her comfort and help her relax—it can be chilly with nothing on!

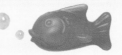

What you need

A baby bath is handy and certainly offers a less-daunting prospect for your baby than the big bath (plus it's easier on your back), but it's not indispensable—a kitchen or bathroom sink will do just as well while your baby is small enought to fit. An innovation from Europe is a slip-free, bucket-shaped bowl that holds older babies securely in the water, mimicking the uterus. And while bath toys are great fun for older babies, you don't need to go there just yet. And when she's enjoying her dips, simply add a couple of pouring vessels or a plastic strainer for plenty of fun.

In it together

Bathing together can be a magical experience for you and your baby. She will love the unique experience of lying with you in the water and feel deeply reassured by your presence; and enjoying skin-to-skin contact while the warm water ripples gently over you is immensely relaxing for you both. Dads in particular may enjoy such bath time closeness and find it a perfect way to bond. And under supervision, older siblings may be thrilled to share a bath with their baby brother or sister.

Too clean?

For young babies with little chance to get dirty, a daily bath isn't necessary. In fact, experts advise against daily baths, partly contributing the rise in eczema over the past 50 years to overzealous bathing, stripping the skin of its natural moisture. A bath-time dip two or three times a week, using only the gentlest of products, and daily washing of the face, neck, hands, bottom, and those tricky creases in the neck and armpits will keep her clean enough. Conversely, once a child has eczema, a daily bath with an emollient cream to seal in moisture is thought to be beneficial.

Naturally soft

The delicate skin of babies has a tendency to dry out. If your baby's skin looks in need of moisture or seems itchy, try a natural remedy such as a soothing soak in an oatmeal bath—the cellulose and fiber in the oats soften the water.

One of a kind

Even though all of us share 99.9 percent of our DNA, the remaining 0.1 percent is enough to make each of us unique.

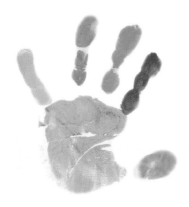

In all our myriad variations, everything we are is determined, at least partially, by what is **written in our genes**. While you may wish for your baby to have your eyes, his father's freckles, and his grandfather's talent for baseball, we all know that it isn't as simple as that.

The first of a baby's cells are created when a sperm fuses with an egg, and this is the cell from which all others will be created. Within the nucleus of each cell are **46 chromosomes in 23 matching pairs**, with one chromosome per pair inherited from each parent. These chromosomes are basically a recipe book or instruction manual for how to make certain proteins, which will form the **building blocks of our bodies and functions**. When examined closely, each chromosome is like a long thin string of beads (with each bead representing a gene) twisted into the shape of a double helix. A gene is made up of deoxyribonucleic acid, more commonly known as **DNA**, and each gene contains an important bit of information about our health and development. These **chromosome structures** are so vast and complex that if the DNA contained within just one human cell was unfurled to its full length, it would measure 6ft (1.8m); the height of a tall human being.

One of the most important pieces of information contained within a cell is the instruction that determines gender, and whether your baby is going to be a **boy or a girl** is "decided" by the father. Each egg or ovum (female reproductive cell) contains within it an X sex chromosome, while each sperm (male reproductive cell) can contain either an X or a Y chromosome, in roughly equal measure. So, it is simply a question of which of these sperm meets the egg first that will determine whether your baby is XX (a girl) or XY (a boy). Theoretically these outcomes each have a **50 percent chance**, just like a coin toss, and indeed the world sex ratio does remain roughly even, but a few more boys are born each year than girls (about 51 percent at this

Your parents would have to have another 1,000,000,000,000,000 babies to stand a chance of having another you.

point in time). Some scientists theorize that this is due to the fact that Y-chromosome sperm are a little smaller and therefore may simply be able to get to the egg faster, but the **lifestyle** of the baby's parents may also have an effect. One study revealed that women who eat cereal for breakfast every morning are more likely to conceive a boy than non-cereal eaters (59 percent, as opposed to 43 percent), but whether this is related to the cereal or some other common factor is unclear. We all know a family who has a lot of daughters and no sons, or vice versa, but it is interesting to note that, in fact, at the moment of conception they have the same 50–50 chance as everyone else.

Your baby's genes will decide his other **physical characteristics** too, such as blood type, eye color, height, and whether he will or won't develop certain health conditions. They also influence **behavioral characteristics**, such as his talents and intelligence, but which gene he will inherit and which trait he will express will depend on a number of factors. Every person inherits two versions of each gene, and in some cases one of the pair will be dominant and one recessive. So, in the case of **blood type**, A is dominant over O. If you are AA (if both your parents had type A blood) and your partner is AO, your baby will definitely have type A blood because even if she took an A from your side and an O from your partner (to become AO), the A would be expressed as it is dominant. The only way to end up with O blood is to inherit an O from each parent, therefore becoming OO. Other examples of **dominant traits** include dark hair (which is dominant over other hair

colors), brown eyes (which dominate other eye colors), and dimples dominate over no dimples. It isn't always straightforward: parents who both have blue eyes can still produce babies with brown or green eyes, since many genes are required to make the black and yellow pigments needed for darker eyes. For a **recessive gene** to appear you need two copies—one from each parent, otherwise it will **skip generations** until it meets a match.

To complicate matters further, not all traits are decided by one gene. Tongue rolling and freckles, for example, are decided by a single gene, but other traits such as skin color, height, and body mass are thought to be contributed to by **a number of different genes**. Research into the field of genetics is ongoing, particularly in medical history.

Identical twins share 100 percent of their genes. Fraternal siblings share 50 percent of their genes.

In many of these cases, however, there is also some interplay with the environment that can affect these built-in blueprints. As diet improves in each country, so heights increase among the population.

In the same way, what is written in your baby's genes is only half the story—there may be many **lifestyle and external influences** that will affect how he develops. This is why it is important to give your child the best start in life you possibly can in terms of care and nutrition, because even the best laid plans can go awry if they are not given the right conditions for growth. With all the wonderful variety of human life, it is one of the most exciting privileges of parenthood to watch your baby become his very own person, familiar in so many ways, but also **unique**.

Times for
togetherness

Your baby is up for anything as long as it's with you so it's good to know there are plenty of things that you can do together that can stimulate you both, while all the time strengthening your bond.

Bonding with your baby enables you to understand and interpret her needs better. Your relationship with her is key to her early cognitive and social development; it forms her first model of a loving relationship, and contributes to her sense of security and self-esteem.

Spending every day with your baby can seem daunting, but she is portable and adaptable so don't feel the walls have closed in on you. Babies constantly soak up stimuli from the world around them, and the greater variety of things you do together the more experiences you are opening her up to.

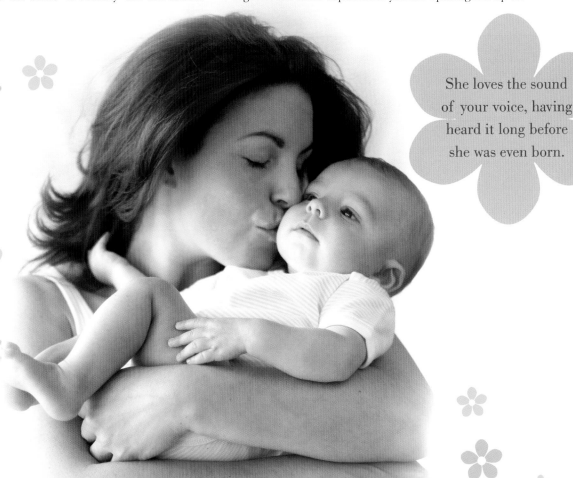

She loves the sound of your voice, having heard it long before she was even born.

Tummy time

About one minute on her tummy three times a day will build up your baby's strength. Rub her back and talk to her, or even put her on your own tummy so that you are face to face.

Nature buddies

Introduce your baby to the great outdoors with picnics in the park, walks along a river, or regular time in the backyard. Set out a blanket under trees and gaze together at the rustling leaves and passing clouds.

The loving touch

Touch is very important to your baby. Holding her skin-to-skin actually has a positive effect on her growth and development, so both parents should spend time cradling and stroking baby to let her get used to your differences.

Carry on

Babies find being held by their parents reassuring, and wearing her in a front-pack baby carrier in the day teaches her valuable information about routines. In turn, you will find it easier to stay in touch with her needs.

> Eye contact is one of the most meaningful forms of communication. Let your baby study your face—memorizing it will be one of her first intellectual developments.

Cultural catch-up

While your baby is still tiny, don't miss the chance to stay in touch with the outside world. Pop your little one in the front pack or carriage and head off to the local museum for the latest exhibition; or check out mom-and-baby daytime movies at the local theater to keep abreast of the latest releases.

Brothers and sisters

Older siblings will love helping you to bathe your baby, and maybe even sharing favorite toys and books. Depending on their age they might also like to cuddle her, give her a bottle, or even have try burping her.

Get involved

Sign up for a mother-and-baby class—there are dozens to choose from, including baby yoga and massage, music get-togethers, fitness and swimming sessions, stroller walks in local parks, and even salsa baby groups and mom-and-baby zumba! In addition to being highly stimulating for you both, enrolling in a class is the perfect way to meet other new moms.

Day-tripper

As your confidence grows, why not go farther afield and make a day of it? This is the perfect time to get on a train or in the car and go somewhere new; or recruit a couple of friends and head off for the beach, visit a historic site, or check out a country fair.

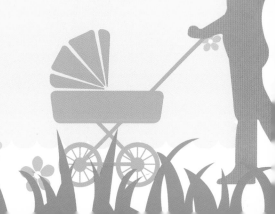

Good days, bad days

Having a baby turns your world upside down, and life will never be the same again—and this is a good thing. But, as with any period of transition, the road can be a bumpy one.

New parenthood is often portrayed as a time of unparalleled joy—contented baby and doting parents cocooned in a blissful bubble. Yet this picture-perfect image omits a large chunk of the day-to-day reality: physical and emotional vulnerability, hormonal swings, discomfort, exhaustion, and the awesome responsibility of looking after a tiny baby. This postpartum period tends to be one of high emotion, where feelings are intense and moods swing dramatically, and studies demonstrate how marital happiness can dip. Adjusting your expectations and seeing parenthood as a process can ward off feelings of inadequacy and help you accept the not-so-smooth along with the truly marvelous.

A challenging time

The preparation, emotionally, physically, and mentally, that people put into other major challenges, such as running a marathon, is often neglected by parents-to-be. Giving yourself a reality check about the challenges you face and preparing for the whole range of feelings you'll encounter arms you to deal with them; so in the time before your due date, pay attention to your relationship and well-being, and put in place coping strategies. Once baby arrives, a recognition that you're both taking the stress engenders a mutually supportive environment, rather than one in which you're competing for "time off." Good communication is vital. Most experts agree that happy parents make for a contented, emotionally connected child.

Share the load

The good days in life should outnumber the bad ones, but if the balance shifts the other way, you need to reach out and talk to someone who can help. Support from a whole network of individuals is pivotal now. Most likely you'll encounter many offers: don't hesitate to say yes—this isn't an admission of failure! And as independent adults it's often hard to ask for help, but people like to help.

There are numerous ways the load can be lightened: grandparents can provide homemade fare, watch baby while you sleep or shower, and help

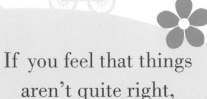

If you feel that things aren't quite right, listen to your gut and talk to your partner or doctor.

with shopping or household chores; partners can share bottle-feedings, stay up with crying baby while you sleep, and take over kitchen duties for a few weeks. New parent groups are a lifesaver, too, offering readily available friends in the same boat, willing to discuss the nitty-gritty of parenting.

A case of baby blues?

The first few days after your baby is born are a time of huge hormonal flux. The result being that you might feel tearful, irritable, tired, and/or miserable. Such a reaction to birth is incredibly common—over half of new mothers experience these "baby blues." Such feelings peak, on average, between three and ten days after the birth and then disappear. If you experience such feelings for more than two weeks, talk to your doctor or a mental-health professional.

A friend in need?

It's not always easy to look at a list of symptoms and spot those people suffering from postpartum depression, but there are signs you can look for in your new-mom friends and their partners. Here are some warning signs:

* Crying fairly often for no obvious reason.
* Neglecting physical appearance, such as not changing clothes or appearing to be unwashed.
* Having difficulties bonding with their baby.
* Being unable to see the funny side of things.
* Having lost any sense of time—always being late or just missing meetings you've arranged or not knowing when they last did something (15 minutes ago or three hours?).
* Worrying excessively about their baby to the extent where they think something is wrong and can't be reassured.

Could it be something more serious?

What happens if you're still feeling exhausted, sad, unable to sleep, or anxious a month or so after your baby's born? You may be experiencing postpartum depression. And you wouldn't be alone—as many as one in six new moms has an episode of postpartum depression; and dads aren't immune to depression either (see pages 144–145). The six-week checkup is a good moment to discuss mental and physical concerns you have with your doctor. If your doctor thinks you are suffering from postpartum depression, getting prompt treatment can help enormously.

Someone with postpartum depression won't be experiencing all of these feelings all of the time, but they will be feeling overwhelmed by such emotions:

• unable to cope • anxious • irritable • guilty • excessively tearful • lonely • lacking concentration • a sense of hopelessness • lost sense of humor • generally feeling miserable.

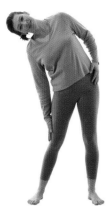

Getting back in *shape*

Confronting your post-pregnancy body in the mirror can be disheartening—a flabby tummy, loose skin, and boobs that are achingly large. You might wonder if you'll ever get your body back. But the good news is yes, you can—it's just one step at a time.

It took 40 weeks for your body to prepare for birth and so is likely to take a while for it to recover fully. Jumping from the labor ward to the treadmill can be damaging, because your muscles first need to heal from the trauma of birth. Gentle is best, for you and for your baby, especially since you now have disturbed nights, a new routine, and possibly breast-feeding to contend with. There are simple things you can do immediately after birth, and after your six-week checkup you can gradually start real exercise.

Regular exercise also boosts your mood and self-esteem, strengthens and tones tired and overstretched muscles, and helps you feel like yourself again.

FROM DAY 1

Work that pelvic floor

All new moms can begin exercising their pelvic floor muscles pretty much right away—regaining strength here will help avoid urine leaks now and later on. And it doesn't matter if you didn't really get around to doing Kegel exercises during pregnancy either, you can make up for it now. Squeeze the muscles for a count of three, then relax for three—repeat ten times, gradually increasing the number of squeezes as you regain strength. Try to do them at a set time, such as during a feeding, so they become a routine and regular part of your day.

FROM WEEK 1

Get those legs walking

Start walking around as soon as possible—simply getting out in the fresh air lifts your mood, and walking works muscles in your legs, buttocks, abdominen, arms, and shoulders, and also boosts your circulation. Pushing the weight of the carriage gives you an extra workout (power strolling makes the most of this, see opposite), and it's easy to build into your day—go to the park, around residential streets, or to nearby stores. Make a conscious effort to go the long way if you can, and try to walk instead of taking the car.

JOIN THE CLUB

If you want company and motivation, go to a mom and baby exercise class. There are usually plenty to choose from, including baby carriage/stroller exercise groups where moms get together to push their children in strollers through parks and open spaces (power strolling). Other specifically post-pregnancy classes don't always involve babies, but if you can time it for when someone can babysit, it can be a great opportunity to meet local moms, shift a bit of weight, and energize your mind and body.

BOUNCING BOSOMS

If you're breast-feeding, try to exercise after feeding your baby or express before you exercise, since full breasts may make you uncomfortable. Some studies have found that lactic acid can alter the taste of breast milk after exercise, but only after a very strenuous workout, so stick with mild exercise for now.

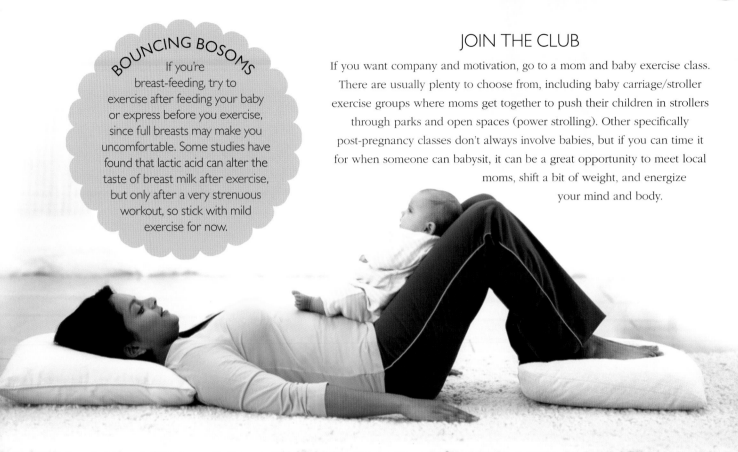

FROM WEEK 6

Swim into shape

It's best not to swim for the first six weeks after your baby is born because there is an increased risk of infection during this healing time. But after that, swimming is a wonderfully supportive way to get into shape. Many pools offer postpartum and baby swimming classes—ask your pediatrician if your baby is old enough and healthy enough to go in a public pool.

FROM WEEK 12

Step up to a new level

Once you've passed the 12-week mark you can try gentle aerobic exercise as well as weight-bearing exercises. Use slow, controlled movements, starting with very low weights (soup cans are perfect and are often already in your home), or go to a gym and ask them to advise you on a postpartum regimen. Yoga and Pilates are excellent for rebuilding abdominal strength and gradually flattening out your tummy, as well as tightening your pelvic floor, regaining good posture, and strengthening your upper body to help you easily lift and carry your new (and rapidly growing!) baby. Always tell instructors that you have recently had a baby.

Natural born *worriers*

A little bit of worrying is not a bad thing for a new parent since it keeps you on the ball: the trick is not to lose perspective.

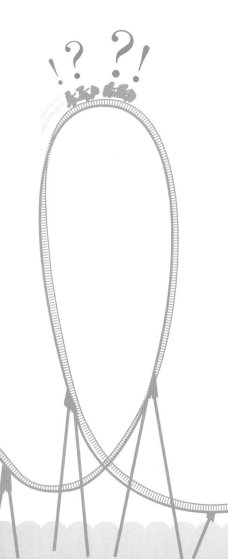

Are you freaking out about every little thing? Scared you are the only one? Relax, you aren't. Go to any online parenting or pregnancy forum and, amid the joys of parents, you will find a litany of worry and fear. It's enough to send anyone's stress levels soaring.

Room temperature, bath temperature, your baby's temperature, the occasional glass of wine you had while you were pregnant, that glass you had just before you breast-fed your baby, the amount of time you hold him, and the amount you talk to him. These are just some of the things new parents stress about. And then there are the really big worries: dropping him, falling down the stairs with him, letting him slip in the bath, loving him enough; and what if he stops breathing at night, gets sick, or develops autism?

Many women worry about changing relationships—will their partner feel left out? Will they be able to love their new baby?

You may feel like you are **scaring yourself senseless** by letting your mind reel like this, but be reassured that worry, pregnancy, and parenthood go hand in hand. A 2003 study suggested that 65 percent of new parents find themselves obsessing about potential harm to their babies. And, in fact, as any new parent will tell you, pregnancy itself is just the start of a lifetime of worry. But the flip side is, it is also the start of an incredibly rewarding two-way relationship, and **worry is just a necessary facet of parental love**.

So, worrying in new parents is common. But why do we do it? According to a study published in *Neuroscience and Biobehavioural Review*, 2011, scaring yourself as a new parent may in fact be **an evolutionary hangover** from our ancient past, when pregnancy and early childhood—vulnerable times even today—were positively hazardous. In those days, very real threats came from infectious disease, violence, and accidents. Some psychologists suggest that our **brains and hormones change during parenthood** to make us vigilant in a way that will protect our babies; although occasionally in the modern day this can slip into overdrive, causing clinical anxiety.

Every parent feels their baby is special, but as far as nature goes human babies really are. No other animal devotes as much energy and time to an individual offspring. The sheer amount of effort we invest in our children means that each one is precious, so it makes sense that we would evolve **strategies to protect them**.

Modern-day studies of hunter–gatherer tribes show that disease is one of the greatest threats to babies. A 2007 study of a traditional Venezuelan tribe showed the death rate due to "congenital problems," many of which develop in pregnancy, and disease in newborns was 30 percent each. If these societies are reflective of our ancestral way of living, then **our parental drive to worry is not misplaced**.

Behavioral changes seen in pregnant women the world over, such as nesting and fussing about food and cleanliness, (see pages 88–89), may occur for good reason: to protect the unborn child from pathogens. Likewise, studies suggest that pregnant women may steer clear of unhealthy-looking individuals, possibly to avoid catching anything harmful.

But what's the response to worried moms and moms-to-be? "It's hormones!" is a common refrain on online forums. Indeed there may be truth to this. Worry can cause levels of the **stress hormone cortisol** to rise; but, in moderation, this is not necessarily a bad thing—it might even make you a better parent. New moms with high levels of cortisol have been shown as more likely to recognize their babies from smell alone; and there are suggested links between a mom's cortisol levels and her responsiveness to her baby's cries. In fact, worrying may be a cornerstone of a natural **biological feedback loop of love**. New parents worry more, so take steps to protect their little ones, and in return they get cute bonding behavior, which elicits love. The emotional rewards they get from their child mitigates their heightened state of worry spiraling out of control.

But can your stress harm your baby? Yes—sustained high levels can affect a pregnancy, for example by increasing the risk of a premature birth. Stress hormones, such as cortisol, appear to cross the placenta, and some studies suggest that babies born to highly stressed mothers may be affected in childhood, particularly by anxiety and attention disorders.

A 2009 Chinese study lauded the soothing effects of music on pregnant women being treated for anxiety in the hospital.

So how can you keep your natural inclination to worry to manageable levels? Parenting and health websites suggest you seek help from family and friends, join parent and baby groups to share your worries, go for walks, get physical exercise, listen to calming music, and sleep when you can.

But remember, a bit of worry may just be **nature's way of preparing you for parenthood**. Be reassured that your body and your little one have evolved to do this. And in the modern day, many of the threats of our ancestral past are vastly reduced, and our health-care systems are better equipped than ever to deal with any problems that may arise.

So, when you check that your sleeping newborn is still breathing for the twentieth time, take a deep breath and try to relax in the knowledge that **worrying is completely normal**. Don't stress about getting stressed.

The magical
three-month mark

Just when you think you know your baby, she changes—that's what makes being a parent such a thrilling journey. At three months she is an infant not a newborn, and this brings many exciting changes that will make your life together even more enjoyable.

Your baby is growing up

Your baby will now be playing and interacting more with you. The parietal lobe in her brain is developing rapidly, enabling object recognition and hand–eye coordination. She will also begin to understand cause-and-effect, for example she'll enjoy moving a rattle to make a noise.

She will find faces fascinating and will watch you closely. You may be able to buy yourself some extra sleep by attaching a safe mirror to her crib so she can watch "another baby" in the mirror.

Her sense of smell and hearing are developing, as is her ability to process language. This is because her temporal lobe is increasingly active. When you talk to her she will make eye contact and she may try to answer you! Talking to her at this age is essential, since it will have a positive effect on her IQ and vocabulary in later life.

Your baby will recognize you both as her parents and know that you're someone special, so when she sees you across the room, she may get excited and flap her arms.

Physically she will have more strength in her neck and back and she may do little push-ups so she can look around. Your baby will learn to roll over, and since this can happen with little warning you should be extra vigilant when she is on the changing table.

Her sense of touch is developing, too. She will be fascinated by how different objects feel and you may notice her reaching out for things to touch. Stimulate this interest by offering her different textures, such as soft cloth, rough towel, or feathers. Touch-and-feel books are also good for this.

 She responds happily at playtime *Her curiosity is growing*

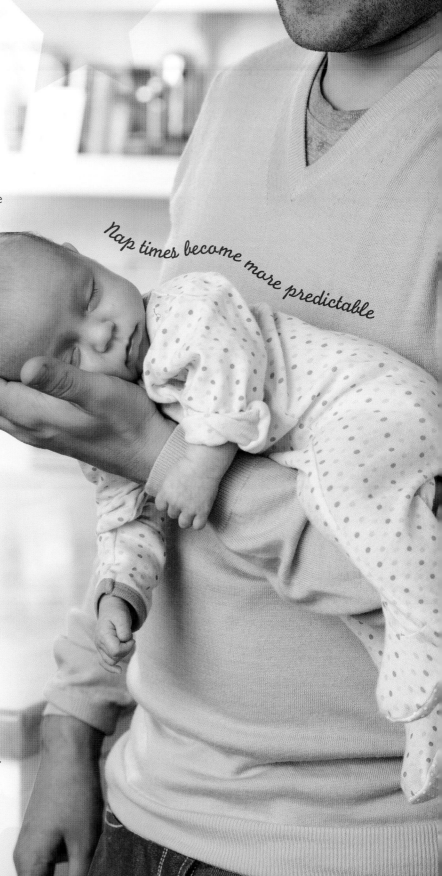

Life gets easier for you

Your baby will sleep for longer periods at a time and some babies start to sleep through the night, or wake up only once to be fed.

Feeding becomes easier since she needs to be fed less frequently and can stay full longer. Her feeding routine is more predictable so your day will become easier to plan.

By now your baby has developed her own routines. She will be more alert in the day and might want to actively play. Her increased responsiveness makes time together more rewarding for you both.

You will now be a lot better at reading and interpreting her cues, and won't always waste time trying to figure out why she is crying.

Changing diapers, folding the carriage, and putting little arms into cardigans are now second nature and take much less time.

Increased neck strength means your baby can hold her head up, making her easier to carry.

You are finding your feet as a parent, and things definitely seem easier. But your baby changes fast and new issues constantly arise. View these changes as part of your parental challenge, and a sign that your baby is thriving.

Nap times become more predictable

You are slowly finding a routine

sleep

* 10–11 hours sleep at night, waking two or three times for a feeding.
* Three daytime naps, totaling five hours.

food

* Needs about seven or eight breast-milk or formula feedings each day.
* Still not ready for solids.

teeth

* May cut first bottom tooth around now.

what a giggle

* Engages with squeaks, giggles, noises, and, in the coming months, belly laughs.
* Smiles for familiar people.
* Watches faces closely, responding to and mimicking expressions.

on the move

* Lifts head and shoulders when on front.
* Soon may roll over from tummy to back.
* Bears weight on his legs when supported upright.

I can...

* Bring my hands together and grasp them tightly.
* Bat at toys and occasionally grab a toy.
* Watch moving objects 5 in (20 cm) away.

my world

* Reassured by routines and the familiar.
* Interacts more, "talking" to Mom and Dad with gurgles and coos, when face up close.
* Has different cries for different needs and uses his body, too, to express emotions, whether he's hungry, bored, or wants to be cuddled.

I am 3 months old

Look at me!
I smile and laugh when you play with me, and I'll let you know when things aren't quite right!

As your baby's muscles get stronger and his movements more coordinated, daily tummy time helps your baby to push up and eventually to roll. Getting down on the floor with him spurs him on to give it a try!

Your baby is noticing more sounds each day. He's rapt by songs and rhymes, which help his language appreciation and introduce the rhythms of speech.

His growing curiosity and alertness are fueled by increasingly finely tuned senses that help him explore the world. His sense of touch is especially acute now and he loves different textures and materials.

Your baby is securely attached now to you and your partner, and is noticeably more social, bestowing smiles all around.

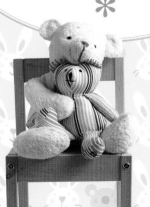
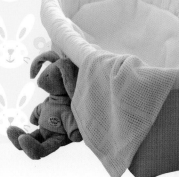

What kind of *parent* are you?

Parenting is about raising a child to be happy, to thrive, and to succeed. But no one said it was going to be easy…

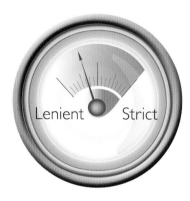

Our notion of "good parenting" emerges from a melting pot of influences: memories of our childhood, observing other parents (real and fictional!), and advice from family, friends, baby books, and health professionals. That's a huge amount of information to process, complicated by some of it being contradictory. Our job as parents is to figure out what's useful and what's not—it's a tough job.

Anthropologists have studied **parenting styles** in order to understand how societies work, such is the influence you, as parents, have. One study looked at parental control in Italian (strict), French (moderate), and Canadian (lenient) families and correlated it with adult values in those societies. Italian society has respect for authority and a strong sense of family obligation, while the Canadians value democratic principles, independence, and negotiation.

Psychologist Diana Baumrind identified three styles of parenting in the 1960s, which still ring true in many Western societies today:

• **Strict, or "authoritarian" parents** value obedience and dictate how their children behave. They have high expectations of achievement and will punish for transgressions to the rules. Not much affection is displayed.

• **Relaxed, or "authoritative" parents** set clear behavior guidelines, but explain why and listen to their children. When rules are broken, these parents tend to reason things through and react in an affectionate way.

• **Liberal, or "permissive" parents** do not set boundaries, instead allowing children to regulate themselves. They avoid confrontation, regarding the parent–child relationship as equal. They are very affectionate.

So, what are the **qualities** we want for our children? Most parents value independence, self-reliance, self-expression, and achievement, and research suggests that the middle way—"authoritative" parenting—produces these qualities. According to one 2012 study, authoritarian parents are most likely to end up with disrespectful, delinquent children. A 2010 study concluded that Spanish children thrived with permissive parents. Researchers attributed this to the low value put on hierarchical relationships in Spanish society. Other academics believe that, short of neglect, **any parenting style works**. Most likely, most of us juggle a combination of all three approaches.

> # Try not to label yourself. You might choose to be strict on discipline, but relaxed about household chaos, and that might all change as your child gets older.

Every culture thinks its way is best, although there is huge variety in how we deal even with the **basic childhood needs** of food, sleep, and attachment (holding and soothing your child). In the US and UK, babies and children often have separate mealtimes, but this isolation from adult society is frowned on in many other countries. In parts of Africa, toddlers are given household chores, whereas Ache children in Paraguay are carried until they are five. In Japan, babies are expected to be content spending quiet time with mother, while in the US stimulation starts early with baby IQ development and lots of verbal interaction.

The best way to figure out what type of parenting feels good to you is to observe your **natural inclinations** and reactions. Where do you think your ideas come from and can you pinpoint specific situations in your childhood that illustrate this? Think about what you can borrow from others: would you like the whole-family mealtimes of your Italian friend and the organization skills of your grandmother? Parenting is complicated by the fact that there are usually **two parents**, even if you parent alone. You might have similar backgrounds, but your partner and his or her family probably have different expectations about behavior, bedtime, child care, and education. **Embrace the collaborative possibilities**: you're making a new family and have the opportunity to remake who you are and want to become.

Let's not forget your **child's temperament**. How might your child respond to the parenting style that feels right for you? Philosopher Rudolf Steiner (founder of the Waldorf education system) identified that children respond to different parenting and teaching styles:

- **Introverted, thoughtful children** may lack body awareness and need a sympathetic approach.
- **Relaxed, quiet children** with inner well-being need a calm, strong approach.
- **Social children** who are distracted by sensations and ideas need friendly interest.
- **Ambitious leaders** with a forceful personality type need a firm approach.

Not every child is so easily labeled, and may vary from one "personality type" from day to day, but it does give you an idea of how **parents may need to vary their approach**.

> # Since every society is constantly evolving, so the parenting goalposts are always moving.

As your child grows, **new situations** will test your strategies as you try to balance your child's needs with those of your family and society. Parenting takes time, lots of sifting through information, and a good deal of talking with your family and friends. And once you think you have it all figured out, your next child comes along and might be completely different. Back to the drawing board then.

Teething *times*

Your baby is born with all his baby teeth inside those beautiful pink gums—and with all the adult teeth waiting below. First signs of teething include gnawing on his fist and soaking tops with drool.

When do teeth appear?

The first tooth usually cuts through the gum around six months, though it's not unusual for a baby not to have any teeth by his first birthday. Equally a first tooth can appear as early as three months. Some babies are even born with one tooth—this tends to be a trait that runs in families. Whenever they start arriving, all of his 20 "primary" teeth should be in place by the time she is two and a half years old.

How will I know?

Common symptoms of teething include irritability, continual drooling, increased chewing (of everything, including your fingers!), inflamed gums, diaper rash, looser stools, a pink cheek, unusual night waking, and crying. A raised temperature or diarrhea may or may not be teething, so keep an eye on it.

Why does teething hurt?

Your baby's poor gums are swollen, with sharp enamel edges poking through, and the teeth twisting into place as they erupt. Ouch! Despite this, many doctors insist that teething does not hurt infants, based on older children's experience of second teeth erupting. However, it's generally agreed that the canines (see opposite) are the most painful to cut, because of their size, followed by the molars at the back of the jaw.

Do I have to start brushing her teeth?

Yes, the twice-daily tooth-brushing chore starts here. You'll need a first-size soft toothbrush and a smidgen of baby toothpaste (the often recommended pea-shaped is more appropriate for five-year olds). Choose toothpaste formulated for this age group, that's fluoride-free, sometimes called "training toothpaste." Kid and adult toothpaste contains too much fluoride for children, as well as digestive irritants, such as peppermint oil.

Will he bite me when breast-feeding?

Not necessarily, but if your baby does give you a little nip while feeding, your reaction will probably be enough to discourage him from doing it again! Offer a chilled teething ring if he seems too distracted to be fed.

When do baby teeth fall out?

At five or six years old, your child will start to lose his teeth—though he will probably be a teenager before he loses all his "deciduous" teeth.

In what order do baby teeth appear?

Usually the bottom, then the top two front teeth (incisors) appear first, closely followed by the teeth on either side (lateral incisors). After a break of a couple of months, the lower molars come in followed by the upper ones. Next to erupt at around 16–18 months are the lower and upper canines (the vampirey ones), followed finally by the lower and upper back (second) molars, from two to three years old.

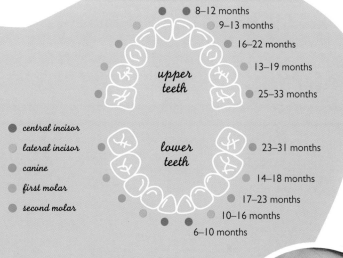

- 8–12 months
- 9–13 months
- 16–22 months
- 13–19 months
- 25–33 months

upper teeth

- central incisor
- lateral incisor
- canine
- first molar
- second molar

lower teeth

- 23–31 months
- 14–18 months
- 17–23 months
- 10–16 months
- 6–10 months

Top 5 teething soothers

Toys and teethers

Keep silicone teethers in the refrigerator, ready to cool and soothe sore gums. Chewing on toys with knobby textures will help teeth cut through.

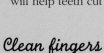

Chilled food

It's dangerous for your baby gnaw on chilled or frozen foods of any kind—he may bite off chunks, which are a choking hazard.

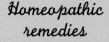

Clean fingers

His or yours! Baby will chew happily on your fingers, and you can also press or rub his gums to alleviate discomfort.

Teething gel

If your baby is over four months, you can apply a smear of teething gel onto sore gums. Teething gels contain a mild local anesthetic and antiseptic that last for about 20 minutes on each application. Ask your doctor how often to use these products.

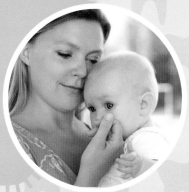

Homeopathic remedies

Made with camomile, these can be rubbed onto sore gums as powders or dissolved in boiled cooled, boiled water and given to baby on a spoon. Check with your pediatrician before using homeopathic remedies.

How to deal with the
first illness

Perhaps the most worrying moment of being a first-time parent is when your baby is sick for the first time. Equip yourself ahead of time and trust your instincts on whether something is wrong.

First things first

Try not to panic—babies easily pick up on stress and will feel more upset themselves as a result. Even if you don't feel relaxed, staying calm will help your baby feel less upset and help you to assess the situation rationally. Your comforting presence will reduce her stress, helping her body to concentrate on fighting the illness.

Fever

If your baby is under six months and you think she's not well, check her temperature. A high temperature (over 100.4° F/ 38° C zero to two months, over 102.2° F/ 39° C three to six months) shouldn't be ignored in a baby under six months since a fever is quite unusual and young babies can't control their body temperature well. However, most fevers are due to "self-limiting" viruses that get better without treatment.

Other symptoms

A fever isn't an illness in itself, but rather a sign that the body is fighting infection. Don't rely on temperature alone when assessing your baby, especially when she's over six months, when it's more helpful to assess her general behavior. In addition to running a fever, if your baby isn't well she'll probably cry more than usual, and sleep a lot (albeit fitfully)—sleep is her body's way of resting and recovering. Understanding that some symptoms show that your baby is dealing with an illness is reassuring.

Bringing down a fever

Give infant acetaminophen and ibuprofen to bring down temperature and ease discomfort. Always follow the manufacturer's instructions and do not use both medicines together. Note that these medicines do not treat the cause of the fever, so if your child is comfortable, there's no need to give them.

+

Make sure she drinks plenty of fluids to prevent dehydration. Increase the number of breast-feedings if necessary; if bottle-feeding, give additional cooled, boiled water.

+

Keep your child comfortable: do not add layers; you can remove layers if the room temperature is normal and this seems welcome. You want to prevent shivering or overheating.

Do not ignore a temperature
over **100.4° F (38°C)** 0–3 months, over **101 °F (39°C)** 3–6 months

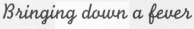

	3|5	3|6	3|7	3|8	3|9	4|0	4|1	4|2	°C
	9|4	9|6	9|8	100	102	104	106	108	°F

Baby's medicine cabinet

Make up a kit at home so you're well equipped for all eventualities:

- a digital thermometer
- infant acetaminophen
- saline nose drops
- nasal aspirator
- teething gel
- bandages
- antihistamine cream
- sterile gauze pads and a roll of medical tape.

A worried feeling?

Can't quite put your finger on what's wrong, but just feel that something is? Don't worry about being a time waster. You know your baby best, and a doctor will respect your instincts.

Good advice

Get acquainted with your local pharmacist, who can provide much-needed reassurance and advice on treatments, or confirm your instincts and redirect you to the doctor if needed.

Time for the doctor?

If she's "out of sorts" for more than 24 hours, it's worth consulting your pediatrician. A visit to the doctor is also needed if vomiting or diarrhea continue for more than 12 hours, or if either is blood-stained; if your young baby has a high fever; signs of dehydration (fewer than six wet diapers a day, dark urine, lethargy, sunken eyes, and a sunken fontanelle); a cold that affects her breathing; a barking cough; sticky eyes; or an extensive rash.

Which medicine?

Infant over-the-counter acetaminophen relieves mild to moderate pain and reduces fever, and is recommended for babies under six months. Infant ibuprofen isn't advised until over six months. Some doctors then prefer ibuprofen since it's more powerful and longer lasting. Follow the manufacturer's instructions on dosage and timing. If a fever responds to medicine, this is a positive sign.

Urgent action

Get immediate help if your baby is having trouble breathing; has a convulsion; an unusual, high-pitched, or whimpering cry and a purple rash; a swollen fontanelle; if she is unresponsive, floppy, or difficult to rouse; or if she is inconsolable.

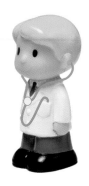

What's up, *doc?*

Since we live in a world full of germs, sooner or later your baby or child will succumb to a bug and require you to play doctor. So, it's time to learn a few tips and build your confidence in recognizing illness and in how to best take care of a sick patient.

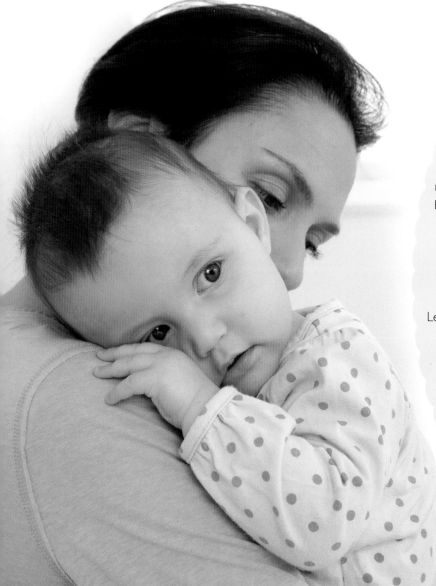

Taking care of your sick child

Stay calm. Assess symptoms without panicking and be comforting.

+

Be informed. Know which signs and symptoms warrant medical attention. Trust your instincts. Don't worry about being a time waster, and call your doctor if you think your baby might need to be checked. If she's under three months, consult your doctor when she's sick.

+

Keep your baby's fluid intake up.

+

Let go of routines. Let your child sleep as much as she needs to, and don't worry about temporary loss of appetite.

+

Always follow the manufacturer's instructions when giving medicine.

+

Don't overdress your baby; put her in a light sleep sack if needed.

+

Keep her room draft free but not stuffy, and her environment comfortable.

My baby's nose is stuffed up. How can I help her breathe easier?

She's too young to blow her nose, of course, but there are other ways to relieve congestion. Saline nose drops help to thin mucus, and raising the head of her mattress can help her breathe more easily at night. Putting a humidifier in the baby's room adds moisture to her environment, or sit with her for 15 minutes in a steamy bathroom to loosen congestion. Make sure she has plenty of fluids, too.

A friend's baby has chickenpox. Should I let my child mix with her to catch it now?

While this strikes some parents as a good idea so that they can control when a child gets chickenpox, or expose siblings together to reduce the impact on the family, doctors advise against deliberate exposure, pointing out that individuals react to viruses in varying ways. While usually mild, chickenpox can lead to complications such as pneumonia and bacterial infections, and, rarely, can even be fatal, so it's hard to advocate deliberately exposing a child to the virus.

Does a cough clear up by itself? My baby has had one for almost a week—should I take her to the doctor?

Although tiring, coughs usually clear up on their own. See your doctor, though, if your baby is under three months or has had a persistent cough for over a week. Consult him or her, too, if your baby is breathing rapidly, wheezing, has blood-streaked mucus, a high fever, or a barking cough with a high-pitched rasp.

How do I give my baby antibiotic eye drops?

Try to do this when she's calm. Wash your hands, then either tilt her head back or lay her flat, gently pull down her lower lid, hold the dropper over her eye and squeeze a drop out, being careful not to touch her eye with the dropper. Let go of her lid so she can blink and spread the liquid. If it's tricky, ask someone else to hold her or swaddle her in a light blanket while you give the drops, or even try when she's asleep.

Patches of dry skin have appeared on my baby's arm and tummy. Is it eczema?

Eczema tends to be red and itchy, and skin can crack and bleed when scratched. If this isn't the case, it's most likely dry skin—the delicate skin of babies is prone to dryness. Keep her skin supple by using an emollient cream in the bath, reducing the time spent bathing, and applying a light, fragrance-free moisturizer.

My baby has a rash—is it meningitis?

Many specific and nonspecific viruses result in a rash, which can be blotchy, raised, flat, spotty, or lacy, often starting on the torso and spreading outward. If she is sick with a fever, then gets a rash, it is probably due to a harmless virus. Specific rashes include chickenpox, fifth disease (bright red cheeks), and roseola (red spots and bumps). The flat rash that can accompany meningitis, known as purpura, is distinctive since it remains purple or red when pressed (use a glass to check), rather than blanching. If this is the case, see the doctor immediately.

My baby seems fussy and uncomfortable. Does she have a stomachache?

Babies can't indicate what's wrong, and even young children struggle to describe the source of discomfort, but excessive fussiness could point to a sore tummy. Look for other signs: is she fussy after being fed, or has vomiting or diarrhea. Causes range from colic to constipation (which can occur when starting solids or changing to formula) to gastroenteritis and reflux. Keep up fluid intake. Consult your doctor if she continues to be out of sorts. If the pain seems severe, get advice immediately to rule out a potentially serious, but treatable, intestinal blockage.

Is ear tugging a sign of an infection?

It can be, but babies also pull their ears when they're teething, overly tired, or just because they've discovered them! If your baby has an infection, you'll probably notice other signs such as fever, disturbed sleep, lack of appetite, cold symptoms, and fussiness.

Illness Q&As

How to make your baby *smile*

A first smile will melt a parent's heart—as the smiles become more frequent, you can try different ways of amusing him.

First beam

You can try getting a gummy smile from your baby when he is just a few weeks old. Wait until he is content and alert and watching your face, hold him about 12 in (30 cm) away (he can't focus much farther than that), and tempt him to return your smile by talking to him quietly.

Babies will smile from birth, but generally these first attempts are just his muscles practicing.

The novelty factor

Above anything, your baby will love gazing adoringly at his parents' faces. But variety is certainly the spice of life, so when an older sibling gets home from school or a friend arrives for a visit, a bit of face-to-face time with the newcomer could elicit lots of smiles. He may also find watching a family pet amusing.

Between one and two months your baby will start smiling in response to environmental stimuli.

Peekaboo

A timeless classic, peekaboo rarely fails to entertain, amuse, and, believe it or not, educate. This game actually teaches your baby that things continue to exist even when they cannot be seen, an important concept known as object permanence. It may also provide crucial training in how to move a blanket off his face. And the sight of your face popping over the back of a sofa or out of your hands will have him chuckling away.

Mr. Tickle

Babies adore being touched by the people they love; it is reassuring for them, and an important part of the bonding experience. Gentle tickling, softly bending and flexing his limbs or perhaps writing messages on his chest with your finger will combine the loving touch with laughter.

Yummy yummy

Another classic: your baby will giggle up a storm if you pretend to gobble up his delicious little fingers and toes. Why we parents feel such a strong instinct to do this remains a mystery, though many theorize our desire to nibble on those digits reaches far back to our mammalian roots (watch how dogs play with their young), and is the start of a gentle education in fighting off predators. Try also blowing tickly raspberries on his neck and tummy.

Acting up

Babies love nothing more than seeing how silly their parents are prepared to look to make them laugh (very silly indeed!). Animal impressions, singing (you don't need to have a wonderful voice), building up to a big pretend sneeze, or salsa dancing with your baby around the living room—it's all in a day's work for a Mom or Dad dedicated to eliciting a beautiful grin and a bout of giggles from their favorite little person.

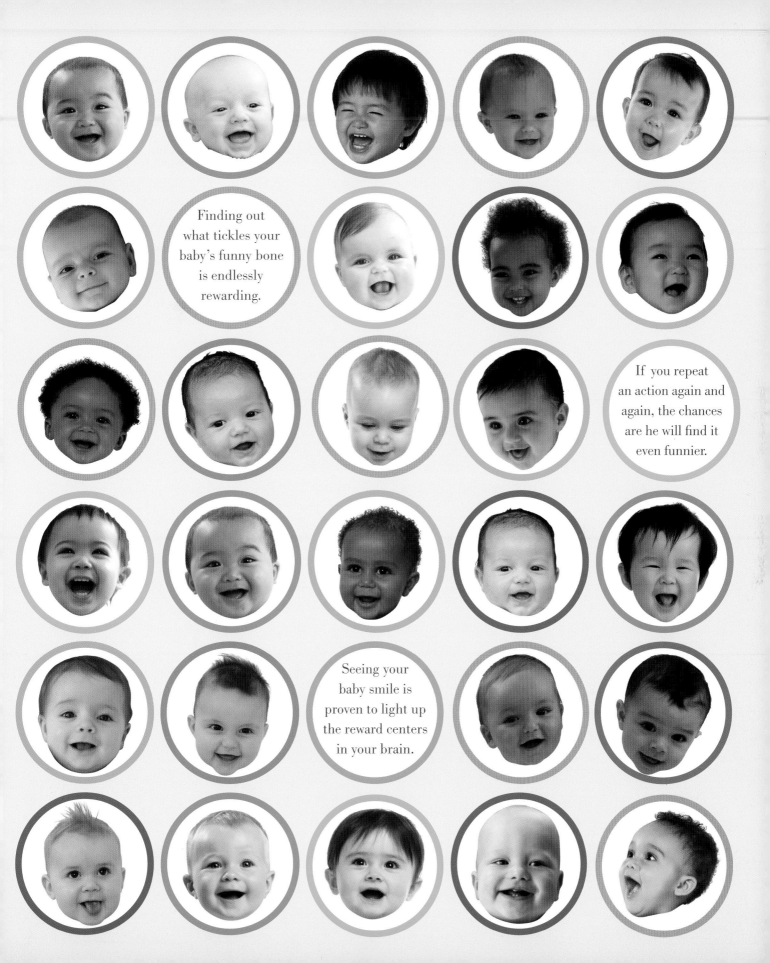

Finding out what tickles your baby's funny bone is endlessly rewarding.

If you repeat an action again and again, the chances are he will find it even funnier.

Seeing your baby smile is proven to light up the reward centers in your brain.

Now I'm stronger, I can reach

Mommy & Daddy

I 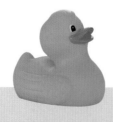 you

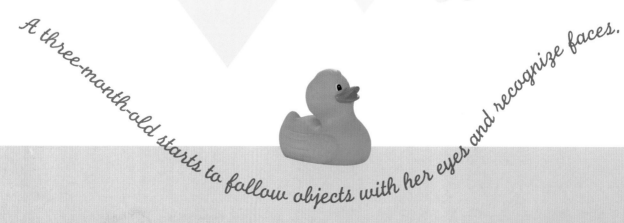

A three-month-old starts to follow objects with her eyes and recognize faces.

and grab what I want.

*Mini-workouts will become
more common—from baby
push-ups and rolling over onto
her tummy to sitting up and
lunging forward.*

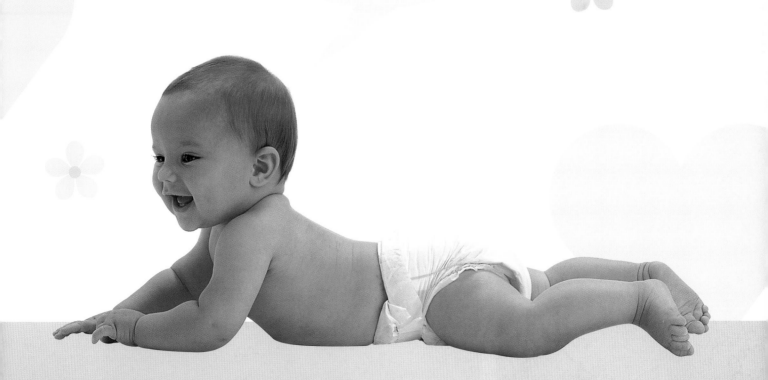

sleep

✱ 10–12 hours of sleep at night, still waking once or twice.

✱ Two naps up to two hours each.

ready for solids

✱ Has one or two small meals a day now—his "first tastes."

✱ Still needs usual milk for nutrition.

✱ Grains, fruits, and vegetables can be introduced now.

✱ Two bottom teeth usually through.

✱ The top two follow shortly, then about one a month thereafter.

new sounds

✱ Gurgles when playing.

✱ Loves repetitive sounds, such as ba-ba-ba.

✱ Babbles constantly, an important prerequisite to language acquisition.

✱ Uses his voice expressively.

on the move

✱ Legs are stronger and can support his weight when his hands are held.

✱ Loves to bounce.

✱ Lunges onto hands and knees from sitting, and may try to crawl soon.

✱ May roll around the room.

I can...

✱ Sit briefly without support—or almost!

✱ Drag objects toward me.

✱ Settle back to sleep if I wake.

✱ Move objects from one hand to the other.

my world

✱ Starts to notice when Mom and Dad leave, which makes him anxious.

✱ Is endlessly curious and investigates everything—often by putting objects into his mouth.

✱ Fearless, and needs more supervision than ever!

I am 6 months old

Look at me! I'm almost sitting unsupported, enjoying solid food, and will soon use gestures to ask for something!

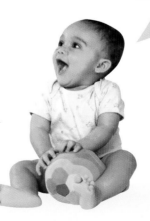

Your baby has a growing self-awareness that he's separate from you which can feel overwhelming at times. A comfort toy or blanket provides a soothing link with the familiar, easing him into new situations.

His personality blossoms as he becomes more expressive. He's more socially curious, too, and interested in other babies: he'll love to "chat" to that "other baby" in the mirror!

Still there! The realization that things exist even when he can't see them is a major cognitive leap for your baby. Hide-and-seek games come into their own now.

Your baby will be well and truly mobile soon and already may inch or roll away from his play area. It's a good time to baby-proof your home.

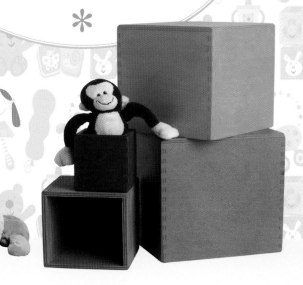

Secrets of sound *sleeping*

All parents can become obsessed with sleep—how much their babies are getting and how much they're getting. Even if you're not following a set bedtime routine, you can still sow the seeds for great slumber times. With patience and consistency, everyone can get some shut-eye.

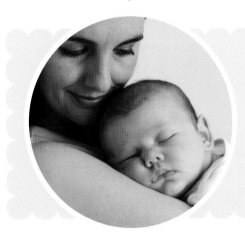

At the end of the day...

Getting your baby into a simple, soothing bedtime routine can avoid sleeping problems later. Keep a regular time for a bath, changing into pajamas, a feeding and some cuddling before settling her down. Put her in the crib while she's drowsy, which will help her to fall asleep by herself instead of rocking or nursing her to sleep in your arms.

Age	Total sleep	Nighttime sleep	Daytime sleep
0–1 month	16 hours	8 hours	various naps totaling 8 hours
1–3 months	15.5 hours	10 hours	3–4 naps totaling 5.5 hours
3–6 months	15 hours	10 hours	2–3 naps totaling 5 hours
6–12 months	14.5 hours	11 hours	2 naps totaling 3.5 hours
12–18 months	14 hours	11.5 hours	2 naps totaling 2.5 hours
18–24 months	13.5 hours	11.5 hours	1–2 naps totaling 2 hours
24 months	13.5 hours	11.5 hours	1 nap totaling 2 hours
36 months	12.5 hours	11.5 hours	1 nap totaling 1 hour

A bedtime routine:

1 *play a quiet game*

2 *give your baby a warm bath*

3 *give her a gentle massage*

4 *change her into pajamas*

5 *read a bedtime story with milk*

6 *sing or play a lullaby*

7 *kiss her goodnight*

Wide-eyed or sleepyhead?

All babies are different and the amount of sleep they need varies. Between 6 and 12 months, most babies have dropped their night feeding and need about 14 hours sleep—breaking down as 10–12 hours at night and the rest in two day-time naps.

Adjusting nap times

At around nine months, she may start changing her nap habits, so you'll need to tweak her routine. If she starts waking up at night, make her afternoon nap earlier and shorter. She'll probably still need two naps a day, lasting up to two-and-a-half hours in total, with a longer nap in the morning.

Waking up again at night

From 6–12 months, even if she's been sleeping through, your baby may start waking up at night. Possible reasons are reaching physical and mental developmental milestones like learning to sit up, roll over, crawl, and walk: teething, separation anxiety, or hunger. If it is hunger you could start her on solids (see pages 198–199).

Sleep training

If your baby isn't sleeping through the night by six months, maybe consider sleep training. Controlled crying—leaving her crying, building up from 5 to 20 minutes before you go in—usually works in a week, but it's upsetting to hear. Gradual withdrawal—when you sit next to her as she falls asleep, slowly moving your chair until it's outside her room—is gentler but takes longer. It's an emotional issue but consistency is crucial, so be strong or you'll confuse and upset her.

A room of her own

According to the American Academy of Pediatrics, the safest place for your baby to sleep is in a crib or similar separate sleep surface. in your bedroom. It's personal choice but, by then—or before—you may be ready to move her into her own room because you're disturbing her and you and your partner want your own space back.

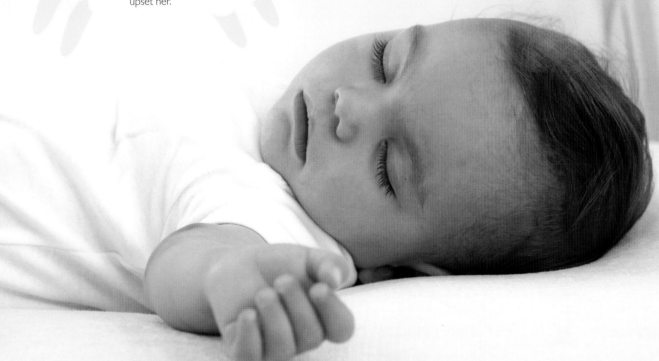

Sitting *pretty*

Over the next six months, your baby's development is amazing.
Physically, emotionally, and cognitively he's making dramatic leaps,
and every part of his world is just so incredibly interesting.

Around six months, your baby will try to sit unsupported. This milestone means he has strength in his abdomen and back, and can now balance. Provide support with cushions, inflatable play rings, and adjust your stroller to an upright position. Limbs will steadily strengthen, ready for attempts to shuffle, crawl, pull-up, and walk.

The ability to sit securely means that he can focus on what he can do with his hands. He can examine an object and pass items from one hand to the other. As his fine motor skills develop he may be able to hold and turn the pages of a board book. Turning and reaching forward is next, as is scooping up

Expand his world

Give him opportunities to explore cause-and-effect with pop-up toys and activity centers with dials and switches. Stack blocks that he can knock over, or blow bubbles for him to pop.

objects, holding and dropping them at will. At around nine months, he'll start to use a pincer grip with his thumb and forefinger to pick up objects.

I get it!

Your baby's understanding and communication skills are changing fast. Development in the frontal lobe of the brain, responsible for reasoning, speech, and problem solving, boosts his capacity to understand complex concepts. He'll discover that small objects fit into larger ones, and begin to grasp cause and effect, so will enjoy pushing toys and shaking musical instruments. He's also realizing that something exists even if he can't see it ("object permanence"), so peekaboo is really good fun for him.

Learning to talk

His babbles become increasingly complex and he's a clever mimic of sounds. He understands more, will listen, and will try to respond by

 Put one object underneath another and

babbling when he thinks it is his turn to talk. He uses gestures meaningfully; when he starts to point, at around nine months, he will indicate exactly where his attention is drawn. Before long, he'll delight you with his first "ma-ma" or "da-da" and is likely to have a smattering of words by his first birthday.

Expressing his feelings

Increasingly self-aware and able to express his feelings in a variety of ways (planting kisses or pushing away), your

 He loves filling and emptying things, so

baby is undergoing complex emotional changes. From eight months on, the realization that he's separate from you can lead to separation anxiety—he may become distressed if you're out of sight. His social awareness also increases, and by 12 months he's likely to enjoy social situations, playing confidently alongside, but not with, his peers.

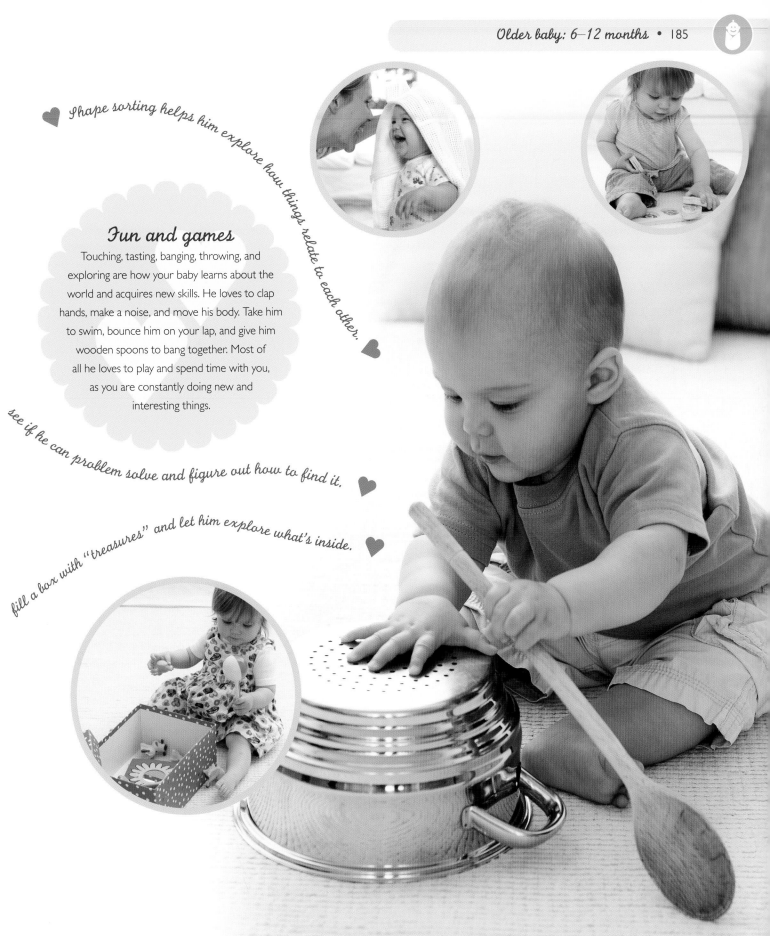

Shape sorting helps him explore how things relate to each other.

Fun and games

Touching, tasting, banging, throwing, and exploring are how your baby learns about the world and acquires new skills. He loves to clap hands, make a noise, and move his body. Take him to swim, bounce him on your lap, and give him wooden spoons to bang together. Most of all he loves to play and spend time with you, as you are constantly doing new and interesting things.

See if he can problem solve and figure out how to find it.

Fill a box with "treasures" and let him explore what's inside.

The sound of *music*

Dancing and singing with your baby is fun, but did you know that music also boosts her all-around development?

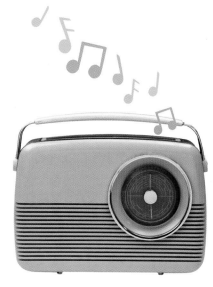

If you have high hopes that your child is going to be the next Beethoven or John Mayer, you should probably start her musical education early. Some babies as young as three months old have shown an ability to match musical pitch, and meaningful singing can begin at around 12 months when parents might even recognize snippets of well-known songs. Children who are surrounded by music and encouraged to use their voices from an early age are usually able to sing competently by the time they start preschool. However, if this important window of development is missed, **musical potential** can literally wither away.

But beyond establishing a basis for natural musical talent, an appreciation and enjoyment of music can also play a pivotal role in developing other vital skills, intelligences, and desirable characteristics. In fact, there are a host of reasons why **making music an integral part of your family life** should be an essential part of raising a happy, healthy child.

> Between birth and six years old, children are developing the ability to understand and unscramble the sounds of their culture's music.

Music plays a role in **wiring the brain**. The process of decoding and figuring out how different sounds fit together—known as audiation—is vital in making the connections that enable the brain to understand and create music. This same process is also believed to improve the brain's ability to understand the complexities and structures of language. Think of the act of singing actually expanding his vocabulary, and even by doing something as fun and simple as making up a song about a daily chore you can actively contribute to this effect. Encouraging your child to **improvise** her own songs, or to fill in the missing words from a well-known tune that you are singing gives her a great brain workout, and will expand her creativity. And, whether or not you can actually carry a tune comfortably yourself, the main thing is to participate and enjoy the musical game, because this way your child will too—regardless of how developed her own intonation.

Researchers have shown that leaning to **move rhythmically** to a beat plays a key part in improving motor skills—there is even evidence to suggest that children who regularly dance and use their bodies to express rhythm are more likely to be able to successfully study and play an instrument. A **good sense of rhythm** is incredibly important in developing coordination, and children who are inactive a lot of the time are unlikely to develop a sense of rhythm and, as a result, will not learn the coordination that improves their natural athletic ability. So, whenever possible you should dance and clap with your toddler, or encourage her to beat out a rhythm, either on a drum or just with a wooden spoon and saucepan. Simple activities such as these will help your child to gain an instinct for rhythm, and encourage her brain to make the vital connections necessary to coordinate eye, ear, and hand.

Music is a well-known **mood enhancer**—most people listen to a relaxing tune when they want to take it easy, or energize themselves during a lull by listening to something upbeat. You can harness music in the same way to stimulate young children. Toddlers who wake up grumpy might benefit from hearing something cheerful or funny as they start waking, whether the tune is being sung by their parent or played on a stereo. And in the same way that babies can be lulled to sleep by a gentle lullaby, young children who are fearful or tense can also be soothed with the right kind of tune. Your natural instinct here is probably to opt for a nursery rhyme or favorite children's song, but classical music can also have a profoundly soothing effect. In fact, it is believed that listening to classical music for a short period twice a day—almost like having a quick "bath" in music—can actually **reduce stress hormones**. This is a good tip to keep in mind for adults and children alike.

Enriching your child's life with music will give her an appreciation of culture.

There are many classes and groups catering to children from the age of just a few months onward that are focused on enjoying music, experimenting with **sounds and rhythms**, and extending motor skills. In addition to boosting musical ability, these classes also work on **social skills** by building confidence, encouraging cooperation, and even sharing, since all equipment has to be passed around. Music may also deepen a child's **understanding of emotion and empathy**; there is evidence to suggest that discerning the feelings conveyed within a song trains the ear and mind to tune in to the emotion behind what someone is saying.

Raising your child in **a noisy, musical home** brings with it a wealth of benefits, and not just for your child; you may find that regular singing and dancing has an equally positive effect on your mood and sense of well-being. Enabling your child to **make her own music** provides her with a vital opportunity to express herself, and in doing so offers you a window into her complex internal life and feelings. Just as the babbling stage is key to learning language, this early stage of music making is equally important. So, next time your toddler is relentlessly whacking your pans with a spoon, try to grit your teeth and encourage her, keeping in mind that one day it may well become a symphony.

One step at a *time*

From the first day of her life, your baby will be working toward her goal of getting up and around like everyone she sees around her. She will do this in stages, one step at a time.

Watching your child grow, grasp new concepts, and achieve the developmental milestones that bring her close to becoming a fully functioning human being is one of the great joys of parenthood. And knowing what her next steps are likely to be means you can help her attempt to master them when she is ready.

Creepy crawly

Even though it doesn't actually get her from A to B, your baby's first step on the road to mobility is learning to sit without help. She will gain control of the muscles in the top half of her body first, so encourage her by pulling her up into a sitting position, and surround her with cushions so that she doesn't hurt herself when she topples. As soon

as she can sit without help she will probably start to lunge forward if you tempt her with a toy. This key physical skill will lead to crawling.

Encourage her to spend time on her tummy several times a day, even if it's only for short periods initially. At around three months she will be able

to hold her head and shoulders up to look around, almost like doing a push-up. She will probably learn to roll over at about six months, and this forms another important set of neural connections. She may also rock back and forth when she is on her tummy; she won't make much progress in a

any direction, but what really matters is that she is gaining crucial experience and strengthening the muscles she will need to eventually crawl.

Crawling helps develop "crossing the midline" skills (using opposite arms and legs) and strengthens the back. Not all babies crawl; many want

Wiggle those toes! Bare feet are best for learning to walk—she needs to be able to flex her feet for optimum balance.

to skip this stage and move right to walking. You can encourage crawling by putting toys out of reach when she is sitting or on her tummy and praising her for reaching for them. Once she is crawling, make a soft obstacle course to challenge her and hone her skills. There are lots of

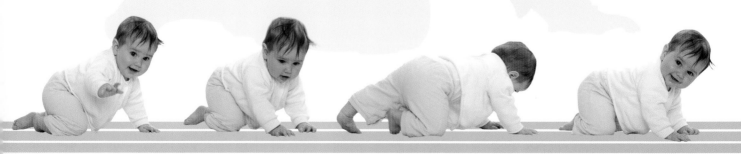

DID YOU KNOW?

Your child may be walking at around 12 months, but it will take another four years before she is able to accomplish the same level of coordination skills as an adult.

Along with your toddler's improving mobility, her fine motor skills are also developing.

different ways to crawl—some babies bottom-shuffle, some scoot along on their tummies commando style, and others move on their hands and knees. Whichever way your baby chooses, she will love the freedom and independence she gains now that she has a more active role in exploring the world.

Get up, stand up

Around seven months she will start to hold her own weight on her legs while you support her; let her gently bounce to build up vital leg strength. Between 9 and 12 months she may start to pull herself up using furniture or your legs; encourage this by putting toys in safe raised positions so that she

has to get to her feet to reach them. Be aware that getting down again may initially be a challenge; guiding her back into a seated position will train her to do this safely.

Cruising for a bruising

Around 9 to 10 months of age your child may start to cruise around the room using the furniture for support. Set up a circuit for her along the sofa and coffee table, for example, to encourage her. Check your baby-proofing now and move anything you think she might be able to reach that she shouldn't. Be prepared for bruises until she is more sure-footed.

Going for a walk

Those precious first few steps can happen any time from nine months to about 19 months. Your baby will probably walk if you hold both her hands from about 11 months and walk along with her, and she will then move on to holding just one hand. But it is important not to rush her—she needs to build up her strength, coordination, and confidence at her own pace. You can encourage

her to refine her skills by providing her with push-along toys, playing fun games, such as walking between Mom and Dad ("one, two, three, wee…!"), as well as giving her plenty of praise and encouragement. One of her main motivations to master the art of walking will be the desire to free up her hands while she is moving. Try to show her how handy this ability will be by giving her something to hold as she takes a couple of steps.

Moving on

Your new toddler will now be carrying things around, moving sideways and backward, and trying running and jumping (though she will initially find it difficult to get both feet off the ground). Stairs will now be a hazard so help her learn how to navigate them—crawling up from the bottom, or turning around at the top and going down backward on her tummy. Always stand behind her. Once your baby has become a toddler the world is her oyster, and she will be eager to explore it. Take every available opportunity to offer her help, because it won't be long before she wants to do everything all by herself.

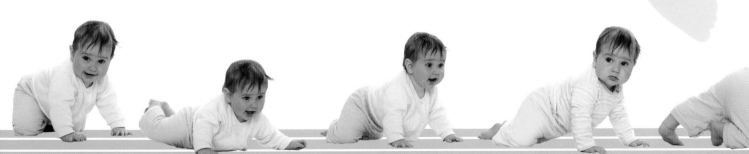

What about *me?*

Being a mom is fantastic (most of the time), but you don't feel like the old "you" anymore. Now, how do you deal with that?

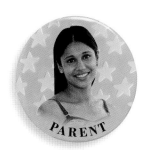

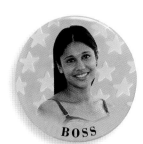

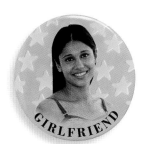

Did you promise yourself: "I won't change at all when baby arrives"? Did you plan to go back to work right away, travel on long-haul flights, go to the gym more often, or spend more time playing the piano? You may well manage all of this at some point, but for most new parents having a baby is a life-changing event. However you liked to spend your days and evenings before baby arrived, whether lying on the sofa or building an empire, things have moved on.

At the very least, you will have **less time to yourself**, and this can trigger an identity crisis. You can't do everything in the same way, so you need to think about what is important to you, and what your priorities are. Of course, being a mom or dad is fantastic in many ways, but plenty of parents also **yearn for pre-baby days**. Finding a way to reconcile the best elements of your new and old life is the best way forward. Having a baby can be a **catalyst for positive change** since stepping off the conveyor belt can give you breathing space to think about what you really want out of life.

When you are expecting a baby, you are the **center of attention** and the first few weeks are all consuming. If you can produce a baby, you can do anything, right? But fast forward a few months and life becomes more routine. It's perfectly normal that your baby takes priority, so your own needs and those of your partner are secondary for a while. But at some point you emerge from the newborn blur and start to think: "What about me?"

If you are on maternity leave, you may not have realized just how much your **work routine shaped your life**. From having a structured week with meetings and goals you're at home with a baby who doesn't fit neatly into an agenda and sometimes the days just seem to stretch ahead. You might find yourself feeling bored and not sure what to do with your time. Or you might find that you enjoy being at home more than you thought, which

Having a baby is the most life-changing experience you will ever go through. You need to reconcile the "old" you with the "new" you.

might be your prompt to negotiate shorter hours or change careers for a **new work–life balance**. How important is your **work identity** to you? If you have always defined yourself by your work role, are you OK to leave that all behind, or do you find yourself telling people you meet what you do, or did, for a living? Remember that all your work skills and interests are still there—they are just being used in a different way for a while. Having less money or losing financial independence can restrict how you spend your time and how you perceive yourself, but you might think the benefits outweigh this.

Your **social life** changes when your baby is young: parenting classes and baby groups introduce you to lots of new people so you socialize during the day, and less in the evening. You may find it harder to maintain old friendships with people who knew you before you became a parent. On a positive note, you might now actually have more time to spend with your partner, family, and friends, and they may see a more relaxed you emerge.

Your changed body may **make you feel different about yourself**. It has managed to produce an amazing baby, but it might not feel like your own for a while, especially if you are breast-feeding or your body has changed shape. If this starts to affect your well-being, then this could be the prompt to reclaim your body and make sure you eat well and add more exercise to your routine. If you walk past a store window and realize that the scruffy, grumpy woman pushing a stroller is you, then it's definitely time to put yourself first in the priority stakes for a while.

Be **open with your partner** and make time to talk about how you both want the next few months and years to be. Life has changed for him, too, and it's easy to lose focus as a couple. Your identity as a **best friend, partner, and lover** is why you both got together, and it's important to keep sight of that. No strong relationship is likely to suffer long-term damage from being put on the back burner for a while, but **keep communicating** about your own changing needs and what you need from each other (see also pages 204–205). Talk to friends too, honestly. Everyone has good and bad days, and openness with other parents is crucial. By sharing your thoughts and concerns, you may find solutions and support, and realize that what you're going through is a **natural rite of passage**.

If you want to try something new, go for it. No need to throw yourself in headfirst—start making steps for the future.

Having some **"me-time"** isn't a luxury, it's a necessity. It's a clichéd phrase but it's a cliché for a reason. When juggling child care, work, and family committments, people (women *and* men) forget to have fun and enjoy life. Make time for something that makes **you feel like you** again, whether you go for a run, read a daily paper, maintain your blog, or have a night out with work colleagues. If you take care of yourself, everyone in your family will benefit, and they will be happy that you are happy too. Being a parent is at the center of your new identity, but it really only enhances what was already there waiting to come out. Working through this new stage of your life brings you to a clearer understanding of the evolving you and makes you the **interesting, unique parent** you are.

JUGGLER

Watch out world, here I come!

I'll crawl over

Crawling activates both sides of the brain at the same time and teaches them to work together. What's more, the brain starts to send and receive messages faster and more clearly as the production of the insulating substance coating neurons rises when a baby starts to crawl.

20 miles before I start to walk.

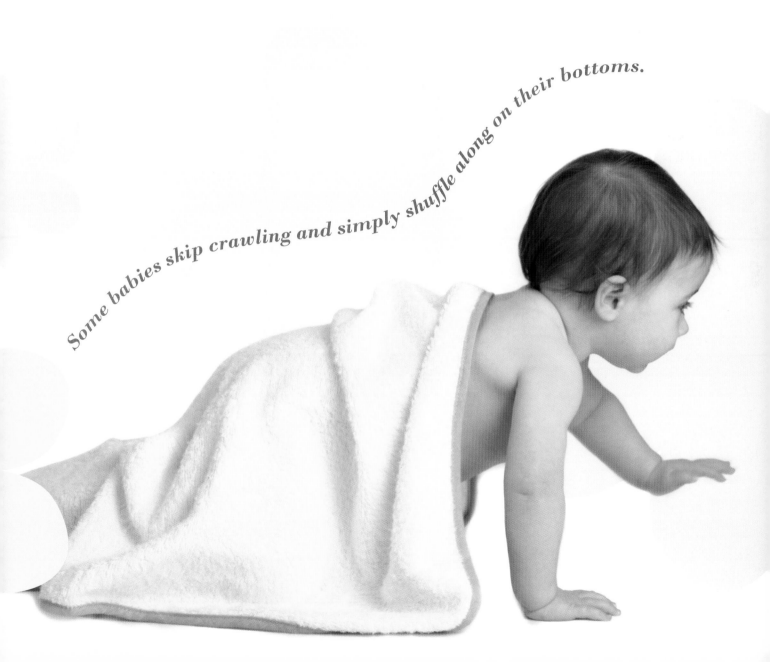

Some babies skip crawling and simply shuffle along on their bottoms.

Don't be *lonely*

When life gets a bit easier, you've got more time on your hands. But don't get stuck at home, there are plans to make and people to see.

Once life settles down and everything gets a little bit easier, you are then faced with the reality that this is now your life. Days follow a set routine, weeks stretch ahead and you must fill them. While some women flourish in the face of this predictability, many can also feel isolated or bored. If you are used to a thriving, successful work life, it can be hard to admit that you are struggling, especially when people will assume that by this stage you are fine. Finding a supportive community of people can help you feel more grounded and connected as you adjust to your new life. Parenting can be a positive time to meet new people, as well as spend more time with family and old friends.

> Routine doesn't have to be just naps and feedings—dates with friends make a week busy and fun.

Nurture prenatal acquaintances

Not everyone from your childbirth or parenting classes will be exactly on your wavelength, but what you do share is a child at the same stage of development, and first-hand practical solutions to sleeping, feeding, crying, and teething problems. Just knowing that other parents are going through the same with their baby can feel reassuring. The families you meet now may also be a great source of play dates, reciprocal babysitting, and even school carpools in years to come.

Join a class

Baby swimming, yoga, and music classes—your child probably doesn't need these skills until he starts school, but parents need baby classes to give the day some structure and to meet like-minded people. Classes can also teach you new ways of engaging with infants that enhance your parenting skills, for example, enjoying the face-to-face contact during yoga.

Keep it local

For many parents, the first time they get to know their neighbors is when their baby arrives. Suddenly, you see your local area with new baby-friendly glasses—parks, play centers, cafés, arts centers, museums, and movie theaters. All such venues offer an excellent way to meet other parents (and local babysitters) and find out what is going on nearby. It's reassuring to explore what your local area offers and to have supportive people nearby, to help you feel part of the community.

Rekindle old relationships

Did you grow apart from some friends or lose contact with work colleagues when they left work to have babies? Now you may have more time to see them, and will have plenty in common with them again. Parents of older children can be an invaluable source of practical tips and seen-it-all advice, and you may find them calmer than other sleep-deprived new parents.

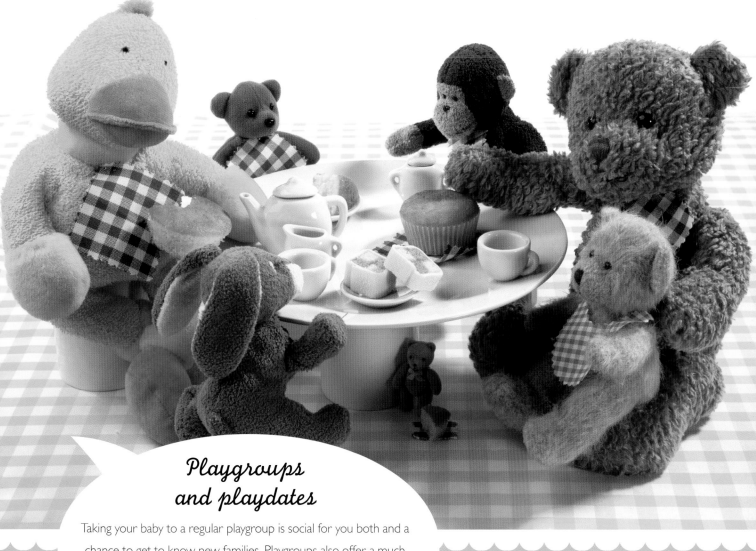

Playgroups and playdates

Taking your baby to a regular playgroup is social for you both and a chance to get to know new families. Playgroups also offer a much wider range of toys and activities than you'll have at home. Reciprocal playdates with friends and their babies, is a great way to catch up in a home setting.

Get yourself connnected

Online parenting forums are entertaining and an invaluable source of advice and connectivity. Whatever you need, there is always going to be someone there to answer you— whether its during a low point during the day or a sleep-deprived night.

Remember, though, that relying too heavily on life online can prevent you from living it fully in the real world. Chat rooms are no substitute for meeting with people, either new friends or old, and any feelings of loneliness you may have will persist if you are not setting up long-term solutions.

Remember pre-baby people

It's tempting to jettison nonparent friends for more baby-friendly company but it's important to remind yourself who you were pre-pregnancy by spending baby-free time with old friends. Make plans to get dressed up and eat out, go to the theater or a museum, play sports, and enjoy a tantalizing taste of the life that awaits you as your child grows up.

Beating the bad *bugs*

Our world is full of germs, and there are, in fact, trillions of microbes living happily inside us. Now, your baby's immune system has to learn to deal with bugs.

During your pregnancy, your baby was protected from exposure to germs by the sealed sac of amniotic fluid. However, after birth she is vulnerable to infection. To compensate, disease-fighting antibodies cross the placenta during the last months of pregnancy to ensure that your baby is born with a degree of immune protection. This **passive immunity** guards against bacteria and viruses in the early months when she's not yet able to make antibodies for herself. Her immunity will be boosted further if you are breast-feeding, particularly immediately after birth when your body produces a creamy "pre-milk" called **colostrum**, which is especially rich in antibodies and other infection-fighting cells. Mature breast milk also contains antibodies.

The routine immunizations that your baby receives at around two months will prompt her immune system to **generate** its own antibodies. This means she has now acquired some **active immunity**, and her immune system will now recognize certain bacteria and viruses, and be able to defend against them in the future.

Once she is a few months old, your baby's passive immunity will slowly start to wear off, and from this point her body has to learn to **fight off** everyday infections, such as colds. An ultraclean home is not essential and the occasional germ and bit of dirt can "prime" your baby's immunity. Her immune system will gradually develop and mature, but in the meatime there are various things you can do to give her an active boost for optimum health, such as getting lots of fresh air and eating fresh fruit and vegetables (see opposite).

Boosting baby's immune system

* Take your baby out into the fresh air every day—this enables her body to manufacture vitamin D, which is believed to prime white blood cells so they are ready to fight infection.

{ *Maintain good hygiene—taking precautions, such as washing hands before eating, will avoid transferring germs to your baby. Remember, though that exposure to some germs gives your baby's immune system practice in fighting them off, so a sterile environment isn't ideal either.* }

* Restorative nighttime sleep plus daytime naps help to maintain a healthy level of your baby's natural killer cells.

* *Avoid smoky places—tobacco smoke contains harmful chemicals that when inhaled can weaken your baby's immune response.*

* Introduce protein into her diet once she starts solids—this provides essential amino acids central to the production of disease-fighting antibodies.

* Eat brightly colored fruit and vegetables while breast-feeding—these contain vitamin C and carotene, which are thought to increase the production of infection-fighting white blood cells, and boost levels of the chemical interferon, which prevents viruses from getting into cells.

Favorite first *foods*

Just when you're into a good feeding routine it's time to start introducing solid foods—and it's a whole new ball game. But rest assured this is a one-way path to a much simpler food life.

Around six months, your baby will need to get his nutrition from additional sources—not just milk or formula. His digestive and immune systems have been maturing and now his body produces enzymes to digest foods such as starches and bile salts. He needs essential extra nutrients, particularly iron—and this is when introducing solids begins. This may at first feel like going back to square one, but soon your baby will be sharing mealtimes with you and enjoying a diet that gives him the energy to move from baby to toddler-on-the-go.

Traditional ways of starting solids

The traditional method of starting solids is beginning with sloppy foods, such as purées or baby cereals, then gradually introducing texture and lumps, until your baby is eating real solids.

Some parents prefer to start with cereal such as baby rice, since it is mixed up with your baby's usual milk so the taste is familiar, and he just has to adjust to the new texture. Other first foods you might try include puréed or well-mashed cooked vegetables and fruits—either offer them on their own or mix them with prepared baby rice. Babies prefer sweet flavors so root vegetables, such as carrots, butternut squash, and parsnips are good, as are puréed cooked fruit, mashed banana, and avocado. Offer each new food on its own first so he can learn to recognize the taste, but soon you can try different combinations. Make sure you keep his diet varied, too; see if he'll eat blended chicken or fish, puréed lentils or legumes. Near his birthday, you may introduce dairy, with yogurt, then cheese.

As your baby gets used to it, thicken the consistency of the food and start to add lumps—even babies with no teeth can chew soft lumpy food. The earlier you do this the more receptive to change your baby will be.

Baby-led starting

Baby-led starting of solids is intended to promote a baby's independence by enabling him to control his food intake. Your baby will immediately eat "normal" foods—no purées— and learn to feed himself.

Offer him soft finger foods, such as small pieces of banana, wafer-type crackers or cookies, well-cooked peas, pasta, or cut-up potatoes, and squash. Lay them out and let him take control. The downsides are that it is messy, and it can be hard to see how much he is actually eating. Yet babies quickly learn how to move chewed food to the back of the mouth to swallow, so the risks of choking are not as great as many parents fear. Sit him up straight and keep him facing forward to help him swallow easily.

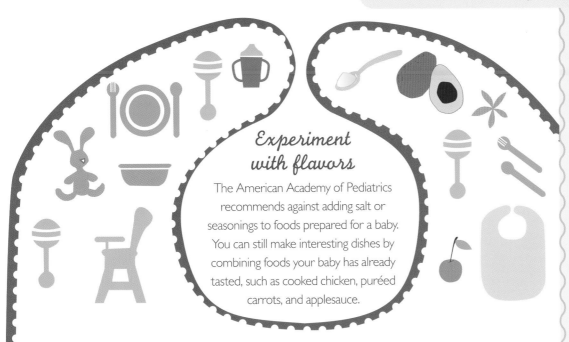

Experiment with flavors

The American Academy of Pediatrics recommends against adding salt or seasonings to foods prepared for a baby. You can still make interesting dishes by combining foods your baby has already tasted, such as cooked chicken, puréed carrots, and applesauce.

Timing it right

Ideally, begin to offer solids half an hour or so before a feeding since you don't want him to be full on milk when you are offering a banana. Equally, if he is starving then his tolerance for trying something new will be limited. Don't be discouraged if he spits it out or even refuses to open his mouth the first few times—it takes a while for a baby to adapt, and you just have to keep persisting each day. Even if he does accept the food, at first he is only likely to taste a tiny bit.

Balance it out

Gradually you are aiming to give your baby a starchy food, a fruit, and a vegetable at each meal, with one daily serving of protein-rich food, such as cooked meat, fish, tofu, or legumes. As for beverages, offer cooled, boiled water from a cup. Fruit juice must be diluted (ten parts water to one part juice) and given at mealtimes only—if he sips it during the day it will damage new teeth, when they arrive.

Freeze it

If you are starting solids in the traditional way, freezing purées in ice cube trays means you can cook in big batches and save yourself time. You can easily defrost a single portion in advance of a meal, or even mix and match a few different foods. Use frozen foods within eight weeks. Reheat only once.

Milk supply

He will still need either breast or formula milk to supplement his diet until he is a year old—after that he can drink cow's milk, goat's milk, or sheep's milk. You will probably drop some feedings, since he won't need to fill up on milk, but he should still have 17–20 oz (500–600 ml) every day.

Foods to avoid

There are only a few things you should not give your baby if he's under a year old:

Salt—his kidneys can't manage it yet.

Honey—it can contain a bacteria toxic to a baby's intestines.

Sugar or artificial sweeteners—they damage teeth and can encourage a sweet tooth.

Low-fat food—he needs a high-fat diet to keep him full of energy.

Foods that are choking hazards—nuts, seeds, popcorn, hot dogs (or so-called baby hot dogs), chunks of cheese, meat, raw vegetables (including carrots) or raw fruit.

Allergies

Allergies are more common if there is a family history of asthma or eczema. But if you suspect your baby has a food allergy, talk to your doctor. Try to introduce foods one at a time, every three days so you have ample time to gauge the reaction.

I've been sucking my thumb

Sucking is a natural action for any baby, and a calming one.

Comforters take many forms—thumb or finger sucking, a favorite blanket, a special teddy bear, a pacifier, or twisting hair around a finger. Such things or actions soothe and comfort your baby whether it's sleep time or a new situation.

since I was in Mummy's tummy.

Hush little
baby...

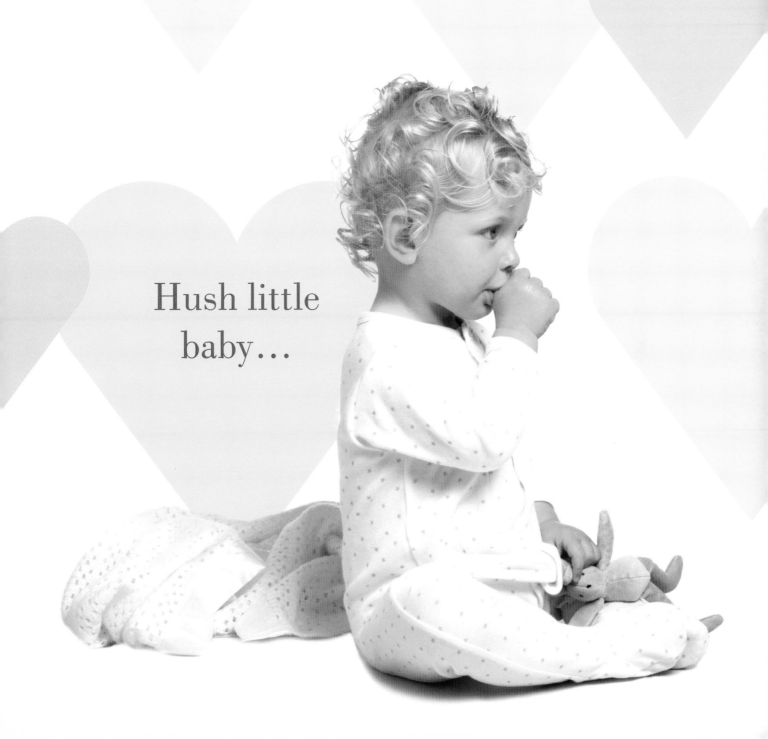

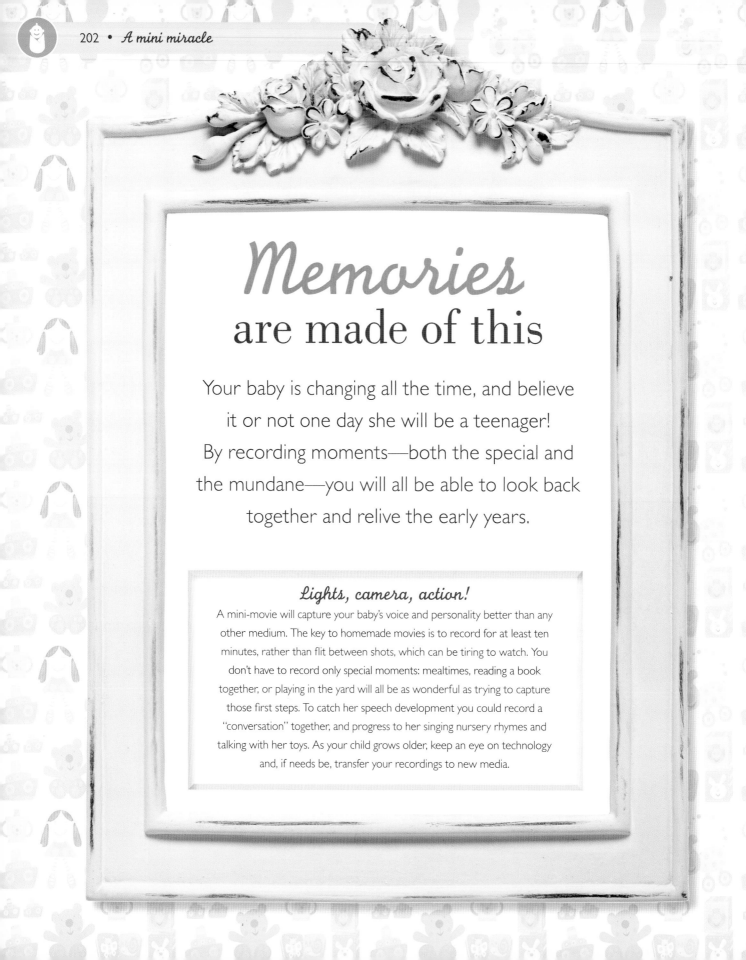

Memories
are made of this

Your baby is changing all the time, and believe it or not one day she will be a teenager! By recording moments—both the special and the mundane—you will all be able to look back together and relive the early years.

Lights, camera, action!

A mini-movie will capture your baby's voice and personality better than any other medium. The key to homemade movies is to record for at least ten minutes, rather than flit between shots, which can be tiring to watch. You don't have to record only special moments: mealtimes, reading a book together, or playing in the yard will all be as wonderful as trying to capture those first steps. To catch her speech development you could record a "conversation" together, and progress to her singing nursery rhymes and talking with her toys. As your child grows older, keep an eye on technology and, if needs be, transfer your recordings to new media.

Baby blogosphere

Many parents-to-be start blogging as a way of sharing news about their baby even before it's born. Blogs are ideal for sharing photographs, video clips, and news with family and friends who don't live nearby. But since online content can live forever, choose what you include carefully. *www.*

Oh-so cute!

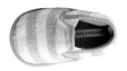

It can be tempting to give away baby clothes or use them for your next child, but perhaps save a few favorite items. Tiny baby onesies, socks, and the pretty cardigan knit by your grandmother will all survive if you wash them carefully, and wrap them in tissue paper. Your child will one day be amazed by what she once fit into.

One-of-a-kind keepsakes

At home you can make a hand- or footprint of your baby either using non-toxic, washable paint, or a clay modeling kit, and frame the results. Pottery painting workshops can help you put your child's prints on ceramic items and there are companies that can make a 3D cast in silver or bronze. Such wondrous keepsakes will remind you of how tiny she once was.

Scrapbook-tastic

Collect your scanned photographs, hospital wristband, and congratulations cards from family and friends to keep in a scrapbook. Add invitations to birthday parties or your baby's christening, bris, or naming ceremony, drawings from preschool, and stick in items, such as a lock of hair. To preserve items longer put them in plastic sleeves first.

Smile please

Easy to look at and more reliable than some modern technology, a beautiful photo album can be enjoyed for years to come. Print out and choose only your best photographs to go in, and perhaps treat yourself to a professional photo shoot, at least once. You can create new albums for each year of your child's life, as well as make mini-albums to give away as presents.

Not just *mom* and *dad*

Your relationship is the reason your baby ever arrived and is
the foundation of your family, so be sure to nurture it, too.

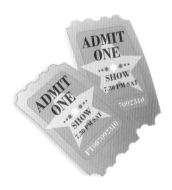

Now that baby makes three, your relationship has had a major shift in dynamics while you both adjust to parenthood. **Spontaneous nights out** and **lazy lie-ins** may be on hold for a while, but many people find that becoming parents brings them closer than ever before. While your new baby will take up lots of your time and brain power, it's important to focus on yourselves as a couple, too, as your relationship is the key to your happy family life.

In the early weeks and months, your conversations need to feature your baby pretty heavily, and that can be very enjoyable and absorbing but can mean that other issues or **just having fun** get put aside. Six months or so down the line after having your baby the early-days haze starts to clear, you look at your partner for the first time in what feels like ages and realize that the most meaningful conversation you've had for months is about who is the most tired. Your **lives have evolved** and you both have different needs and priorities. Even when it's positive, change involves some level of **stress and a period of adjustment** as you both get used to your new roles. If you add fatigue, hormones, and less time into the equation, it's no surprise that many **relationships have bumps** at this time. Research shows a high number of couples separate in the first year after having a baby, so you need to put in some effort to make sure this doesn't happen to you.

You may see yourself in a new way and new aspects of your personality may come out that will have an impact on **how you both get along**. Some new fathers express that although they love being a parent, they feel sidelined in the early months, especially if they return to work full time. A distance can grow between couples since whoever is at home meets new people, has **different topics of conversation**, and there is less time to share the interests you both had. Some mothers feel isolated at home, and become

Happy parents make for a happy family. It's important for parents to view themselves as a couple first and as parents second.

frustrated with the domestic treadmill and grow envious as their partner heads off to work; and the partner going to work may well envy the stay-at-home life. You might think that the person going out to work hasn't had to change their life as dramatically, and therefore doesn't really understand. So how do you handle these potential relationship problems?

Communication is crucial, even when you feel you don't have the time. You may feel that you can't complain given that you wanted this new baby, but it is important to share your feelings. **Keep talking and be honest** with each other. As soon as baby is settled, make time to sit down together and talk before you rush around to tidy up, cook dinner, or go out. Don't assume your partner is a mind reader: you must tell him or her how you're feeling.

Having a baby is a natural point for a **relationship review**. Plan a night together and talk through new ground rules that work for you both. For instance, it doesn't mean the person at home with the baby is solely responsible for all shopping and cooking, unless that's what's agreed. **Share the load** to prevent resentment or misunderstanding from seeping in. Don't get into set patterns: just because your baby is used to you putting him to bed, your partner should take a turn too. This helps to keep your relationship equal.

Becoming parents can **bring you closer**, and deepen your bond and commitment to each other. Talk about your **hopes for your family life** and plan exciting times including vacations, days out, and remember the ideas, ambitions, and dreams you had before baby came along. **Communication and intimacy** are essential to strengthen your bond and to help you deal with any problems that occur. The real threat to a relationship isn't a temporary lack of sex, but a **lack of intimacy**. Strive to preserve this at all costs. Hold hands, cuddle, and give each other compliments. Ask questions about each other's day, and stop what you are doing to really listen. This all helps to safeguard your **emotional connection** and foster intimacy.

Simple, kind gestures, such as running a bath or recording a favorite program for your partner, can make him or her feel nurtured. **Sex is important** too, to reinforce your bond as a couple. If you are feeling too tired or have a flagging libido, it can be the last thing you want to do, but the less sex you have, the less you want, so when you feel ready, make the effort. Switch off the television and share a bath or give each other a massage. Remember that the early baby years go very quickly and relationship difficulties are usually just a phase, so be forgiving of this.

Set aside at least ten minutes every day to sit down together (no television) and catch up with each other's news.

Make time for the two of you as a couple by finding a babysitter and going out regularly, at least once a month, and more often if you are used to having a busy social life. If you don't have family nearby or can't afford a babysitter, arrange **a babysitting swap** with a friend or neighbor. Or when your baby falls asleep, share a romantic late-night meal. If you are tired or are on a tight budget, arrange an evening together at home with a DVD and bottle of wine. It doesn't really matter what you do **as long as you do it together** and remind each other why you were attracted to each other to begin with.

When to *wean?*

We all know the benefits of breast-feeding, but at some point you and your baby are going to be ready to move on. No two stories are the same but there are some guidelines that can make the transition from breast-feeding as smooth as possible.

What you gain

Though it is completely normal to feel a little wistful at first, stopping breast-feeding is a milestone: your baby is gaining independence and you are moving into an exciting new phase together. Now you can reclaim your body as your own and, as your hormones gradually stabilize, your breasts will settle down to a fixed size. That's not to say they won't look different; pregnancy and breast-feeding will change them. But you will know, as every mother does, that you wouldn't sacrifice one second of your time feeding your baby to have your perkier boobs back. So, treat yourself to a beautiful, new, expertly fitted bra—you (and your hard-working breasts) deserve it.

Moving on—how to stop breast-feeding

Timing it right

While the World Health Organization recommends exclusive breast-feeding for the first six months, and then to continue in combination with solid food for at least two years, this timetable won't work for everyone. You may be going back to work, have health issues, such as persistent mastitis (inflammation of the breast tissue), need medication that prohibits breast-feeding, or become pregnant. Or you may just feel the need to stop. Whatever your reason, the timing of when to start solids is up to you. Even just a few days or weeks of breast-feeding are highly beneficial to a baby.

Take it slowly

Your baby should start on solids slowly, initially cutting out the breast-feeding she seems least interested in and then a few days later, phasing out another. Making it a slow transition will mean that antibodies will be more concentrated in the final feedings, and she will be protected as she enters this new stage. A gradual process will also benefit you, since it will help to avoid problems such as mastitis, particularly if you are stopping in the early months. If you need to stop breast-feeding suddenly, you should express regularly (just enough so that your breasts feel comfortable).

Adapt the routine

Depending on your baby's age, she will switch to drinking formula or milk from either a bottle or a cup. Babies who are used to having bottle feedings will accept the change more readily since there will be little, or no, change to their routine.

If your baby is older, the transition may be tougher, but explain to her what is happening and reassure her with plenty of cuddling and other intimate times during the day. Keep her busy and distracted, and perhaps replace feeding time with story time.

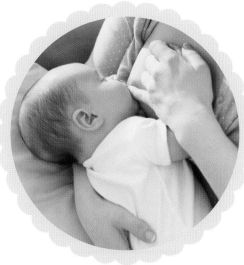

{ In the US, only 36 percent of new moms are still breast-feeding exclusively at three months. }

If you or your baby is finding the transition tricky then perhaps ask your partner to take the lead at bedtime so the issue isn't raised. Your baby may be able to still smell your milk on you at first, which might upset her and account for why she is being resistant to taking a bottle. And try to make sure that starting solids doesn't coincide with other momentous events in her life, such as starting day care.

Stand your ground

When it comes to how long you breast-feed try not to be persuaded by the pressure of others. Plenty of people have strong opinions and very often will be eager to let you know their thoughts—whether it be disapproval that you are stopping or shock that you are continuing into toddlerhood. Don't feel there is a right or a wrong way—there are lots of reasons governing your decision, and you don't need to explain yourself to anyone: your breasts, your business!

Your first vacation as a new family is an exciting milestone, even if you feel a bit daunted about packing two weeks' worth of supplies—and the rest. In reality, traveling with a young baby can be oh-so easy.

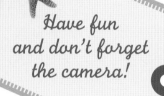
Have fun and don't forget the camera!

Baby's first *vacation*

A smooth trip

For small babies, people are the best entertainment, but you may also want to take a few small toys and books as extra distractions. A change of scenery helps, too—walk around the plane or train, or stop the car and have a quick stroll. Give your baby a drink or a breast-feed or formula-feed during take off and landing to avoid any painful earache due to the effect of pressure differences.

Be prepared

It's a good idea to take a few emergency essentials with you, just in case. Pack some infant fever reducer and teething gel and perhaps a sting gel or antihistamine cream for insect bites. And if your vacation is going to be a sunny one, make sure you've packed your baby's hat, UV suit, sunglasses, and portable sun pod, as well as plenty of sunscreen.

Car sense

Your young baby should travel in a rear-facing car seat in the back of the car; it's probably safer to take your own car seat but it is possible to rent one if you're renting a car at your destination. It's definitely worth taking some window shades to shield your baby's skin and eyes from the bright sunshine and to keep him cool and comfortable.

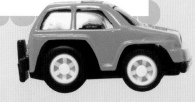

Your baby's skin is five times thinner than yours and contains very little melanin— so sun protection is vital.

All-terrain traveling

Front carriers or slings can be useful for places where a stroller is unwieldy, such as beaches, cobbled streets, or museums. If you're not taking your own travel crib, don't forget to reserve a crib at your accommodation. Your baby's own bedding with their familiar smell will help him settle down to sleep. A universal bath plug will turn a shower into a bath, or, if there's room, bathe him in the basin (put socks over the faucets for safety!).

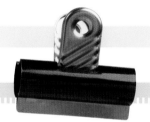

Staycation vs vacation

Vacationing abroad can be more relaxing than you think. A long car trip can actually be more stressful than a short plane ride. Your baby will need the same vaccinations against diseases as you if you're venturing somewhere exotic, so check with your doctor about what you need and how soon beforehand to have it.

Safe in the sun

Babies, like all children, can get hot and dehydrated in warm weather, so you might need to offer extra milk or water. Your baby's delicate skin can burn in as little as 15 minutes if unprotected; it's best to keep babies out of direct sun especially when ultraviolet levels are at their most intense (between 10 am and 3 pm) until they are at least six months old. To keep him cool, dress him in light long-sleeved tops, pants, and a hat, even on cloudy days. Opt for a 30+ SPF "broad-spectrum" sunscreen formulated for children and slather it on 30 minutes before you head outside. Remember his hands, feet, and ears. Reapply liberally every two hours and after swimming. Take a clip-on umbrella or mesh stroller screen for use even on cloudy days. Portable tents or sun pods made from ultraviolet-screening fabric are perfect for the beach, outdoor playtime, picnics, and daytime naps, and usually pack very flat.

Food matters

Breast-feeding is a boon on vacation because you don't need to take any equipment. If you are formula-feeding, you can get travel packs of ready-to-use formula, and carry enough on the airplane to reach your destination. It's exempt from the 3-ounce limit. Extra formula for the trip should be packed in your checked luggage.

Stay at home or...

Deciding when—or if—to return to work is a decision best made when you are not sleep deprived. You need to figure out what is best for your new family in the coming months and years.

If you have a choice about whether to return to work or not, try to delay your decision until your baby is not quite so new and things settle down. You may discover you want to take more time off to be with your baby. Or having planned to stay at home, find you miss the sense of purpose and identity work gives you.

Stay-at-home parents

If you choose to delay returning to work for your child's early years, you won't miss those precious milestones like her first words or first steps. But be prepared for a period of adjustment triggered by losing your financial independence and your career taking a back seat for a while.

DADS AT HOME

More families choose which parent stays at home based on income and who is best suited, rather than assuming it's always the mom.

In the UK, 1 in 7 fathers are stay-at-home dads; this has tripled in the last 15 years.

what are my options?

Family and friends

The major benefits are more flexibility with their time and the low, or no, cost of care. Plus, your child will be taken care of by someone she knows well and loves.

The downsides, however, are that issues, such as wages, costs, food, discipline, and activities, may be contentious. If grandma is sick or on vacation, then you'll have to arrange cover. Other children joining in the child-care setup may also affect and lessen flexibility.

Sharing with your partner

The big plus is that you know your child is always being taken care of by one of his parents. And you avoid child-care fees entirely, which may be a critical factor in decision making.

Although you and your partner are seeing more of your baby, effectively you'll be doing "shifts," so you will both need work with flexible arrangements. You'll need a backup plan to cover sickness or busy times.

Day-care centers

A popular option for many working parents, day-care centers are well regulated and provide a good learning and care structure from trained staff. They're reliable and open most of the year, they are social and fun for children.

Because your child is one of many, she may receive less one-on-one attention, although there are guidelines on staff-to-children ratios. Day-care centers can be expensive, often have a waiting list, and can't always be flexible.

... back to work?

Full-time working

If you and your partner both want to work full time, arranging good child care is crucial. If only one of you goes back, the decision is likely to be based either on who earns the most, or on who'll thrive at home. For whoever returns to work, the guilt factor is sure to rear its ugly head. Acknowledge your guilt (and discuss it with your partner), but remind yourself why you've made this choice and focus on the benefits.

Making part-time work

Working fewer days or some days at home can be an ideal blend of job satisfaction, income, and more time with your baby. Child-friendly options include part-time, flexi-working, compressed hours, or working from home. You and your partner may both prefer to adjust your working patterns and switch to part-time hours; the pluses being you save on child-care costs and you both get to spend more time with your child. Make sure you talk about and agree on areas of responsibility and household chores, so you share the workload fairly.

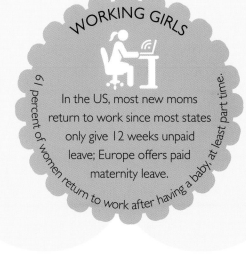

WORKING GIRLS

In the US, most new moms return to work since most states only give 12 weeks unpaid leave; Europe offers paid maternity leave.

61 percent of women return to work after having a baby, at least part time.

Home-based day care

If you feel your baby would be better off in a smaller group or a home environment, then home-based day care is a great option. They are well regulated, offer more individual care, and are a better value and more flexible than day-care centers.

If your caregiver is ill or takes a vacation you must find alternative care. Because this day-care option is in someone's home, your baby may encounter her older children when they come home from school.

Nannies

One-on-one care in your home comes at a price. Nannies come highly qualified, provide balanced meals, organize stimulating activities, and take care of all child-related chores. They can "live in" or "live out" and be shared by two families.

The downside is cost—nannies are the most expensive child-care option. Hiring a nanny makes you an employer; you will have to pay tax, Social Security, and vacation pay, and health insurance.

Au pairs

A low-cost option, au pairs work for pocket money and board only. They can bond well with your child, will babysit, help with light child-related jobs, and may even introduce a new language.

To balance out the low cost, they have no formal child-care qualifications, and can only watch your children for a set number of hours per week. What's more, you need a spare room and ideally a bathroom since they "live in."

The *generation* game

Mutually enriching, the relationship between your baby and her loving grandparents is well worth nurturing.

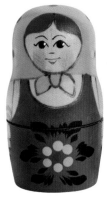

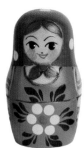

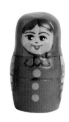

Your parents and your partner's parents may have been anticipating their grandchild for a long time, and doubtless when they finally met him it was love at first sight. This is likely to be one of the closest and most important relationships in your little one's life, and is equally special to his grandparents. You will probably find that the arrival of a grandchild gives your parents and in-laws **a new lease on life**, while your child will be enriched and reassured by their close bond.

Many modern grandparents do not match the traditional stereotype of the the doddering gray-haired couple. People are living longer, continuing their careers, traveling more—and **today's grandparents are busier, healthier, and ever younger at heart**. However, while it might have been assumed that this generation would be too busy with their own lives to have much time for their grandchildren, this is proving not to be the case; in fact, 40 percent of grandparents live within an hour's drive of their families and provide regular child care while mothers work. Even if you aren't relying on your parents for child care, they can be **an invaluable source of support** and experienced babysitters—with the added advantage that they deeply love their charge and cherish the time spent together.

You've probably seen **a whole new side to your parents** since your child was born. You may have found yourself slack-jawed as they produce yet another bag of jelly beans, when you clearly remember that when you were a child you were only allowed candy on Saturdays. They are exercising their privilege of adoring your child without the pressure of actually having to parent him, and the best part of this is that they **often have more time and patience** for him than you. The downside of their tendency to indulge him is that it could create tension between you. Problems arise when your little one starts to think that your rules don't apply, or has new expectations

A Welsh proverb tells us that perfect love sometimes does not come until the first grandchild.

based on what his grandparents allow. You might be trying to get him to go to sleep, only to be told that Grandpa always reads him seven bedtime stories first. If this kind of thing consistently causes difficulties, you should be completely honest with your parents or in-laws and discuss your routines so that they can support you.

However, as long as the occasional divergence from your at-home routine doesn't cause too many difficulties, it is probably best to accept that when your child is with his grandparents, it is their rules that apply, not yours. It may irritate you that he doesn't get to bed on time when they are taking care of him, but the main thing is that they are enjoying his company, and **it won't hurt him to be spoiled a little** once in a while. In any case, his grandparents may not be appreciative of being left long lists of instructions by you. Even if you feel that their methods are a little out of date, rusty, or just different than your own, you should trust them to do what's right for their grandchild. After all, they didn't do such a bad job of raising you and your partner.

But just as you need to stand back to allow grandparents to be themselves with their grandchild, they may need to **respect your way of doing things**, too. You may not appreciate unsolicited advice or constant suggestions from them, and feel it's important to make your own way and be free to make your own mistakes. Beware though of systematically disregarding their advice, since there may be times when they are an invaluable source of guidance when you find that you have no idea what you're doing and are busy wishing that your baby had come with an instruction manual. There's no shame in making use of their years of experience—some of the **essential truths about parenthood never change**, regardless of current thinking.

If you live near supportive parents, try to see them as often as possible, and once your child is old enough, give them time alone with him so they can really get to know each other and have the chance to create their own meaningful traditions and routines. If you don't live close by, make sure you have regular dates via webcam. Grandparents can tell stories and share songs or new words, and in this way your baby will become familiar with their faces and voices, so that when they do get together he will recognize them immediately and quickly feel comfortable. Posting photo albums and videos online regularly will keep everyone in the loop, and, in turn, grandparents can provide a webcam tour of grandma's garden or grandpa's snoring dog to keep them involved in each other's daily lives.

Knowing how much his grandparents love him will build your child's confidence.

Now you are a parent you may find you **understand your own parents more**. You may look back on your childhood, and on the twists and turns of your relationship with your parents, and be able to put yourself in their shoes. It's not hard to see why your mom went through the roof when you got home at 2am, now that you know how deep the love for your little one runs. You are a model for your child in terms of how a parent should be treated, so make sure you are loving, open, respectful, and generous with your parents, so that your child will follow your example. Most importantly, take the time to **nurture this special relationship** so your child can benefit from the precious love and attention of someone who loves him just as unconditionally as you do.

Baby's first *shoes*

Walking is a magical milestone and buying your baby's first pair of shoes is part of that. A world of rain boots, sneakers, school shoes, and party shoes is waiting…

Your baby's feet have lots of growing and developing to do until they reach their adult size, with 26 bones in each of their feet. While they're growing, make sure socks and footies have plenty of foot space for his feet to grow and spread. It can take, on average, 18 years for his feet to reach their final size, with most growth happening in the first three years.

Shoe business

Babies don't really need shoes until they start to walk, and in many warm climates they do without. You might want something to keep his feet warm, and to keep his socks on when out and about, and soft carriage shoes are more than enough until walking starts. Being barefoot is best for the development and growth of his feet, so leave them bare as often as possible.

How to choose the right pair of shoes

According to the American Podiatric Medical Association, toddlers need to protect their feet in lightweight, flexible footwear made of natural materials when walking outside or on rough surfaces. When you are ready, have his feet measured by a qualified children's shoe fitter. Shoes should have space for his toes to lie flat but shouldn't be too loose. They should hold the heel in place and stop the foot from slipping forward and damaging the toes. Bend the soles to make sure they're flexible and not stiff; you can now buy shoes for children with thin, protective soles that allow the foot to move as if walking barefoot. Choose shoes made with natural materials, such as leather, cotton, or canvas, so air can circulate. Good children's shoes will come in width fittings, since feet will change width as they grow. Adorable as some shoes are, don't put the cute factor before a good fit. We don't always remember that as adults (fashion often rules over comfort!), but it's really important to get it right for your baby. Some stores take a keepsake photo of first shoes to mark the occasion, or you could take your own at home as a memento.

Happy (growing) feet

The "bones" in a baby's feet are made not from true bone but a flexible, rubbery material called cartilage, which lengthens as the feet grow. At six months, a baby's foot bones are still mostly cartilage. By three years, around 45 "bone centers" have appeared, making the rubbery foot bones harder. But large zones of cartilage remain, allowing the feet to keep growing for up to 15 more years.

By age 18, the cartilage has disappeared and the bone centers have fused, leaving just 26 complete bones. Hard shoes can constrain a toddler's feet and cause the soft cartilage tissue to develop abnormally, leading to flat foot or other problems. Letting toddlers run around with no shoes on helps their feet grow naturally and normally.

Barefoot in the park?

Growing expert opinion says it's best for toddlers and older children to be barefoot whenever it's safe, because it allows your child to feel the floor or ground and use the natural grasping action of his toes. This will help him develop his balance and will promote stronger, more coordinated foot muscles as well as sending signals from nerve endings on his soles to the brain. Children also enjoy the sensation of different surfaces. Of course, this has to be balanced against not wanting them to step on dirt, dog feces, or broken glass with bare feet. Barefoot at home but not outdoors is probably ideal.

DID YOU KNOW?

A US study cited two-thirds of all adults have foot problems, many of which can be directly attributed to having worn badly fitting shoes as a child.

Over 97 percent of babies have flat feet due to a thick wad of fat in the soles of their feet. Arches develop as they gradually gain muscle.

Some toddlers like to walk on tiptoes, an instinct that helps them develop balance, but persistent tiptoeing may be a sign of muscle problems.

The longest journey starts with a small step.

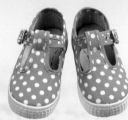

The "bones" in a baby's feet are made not from true bone but a flexible, rubbery material called

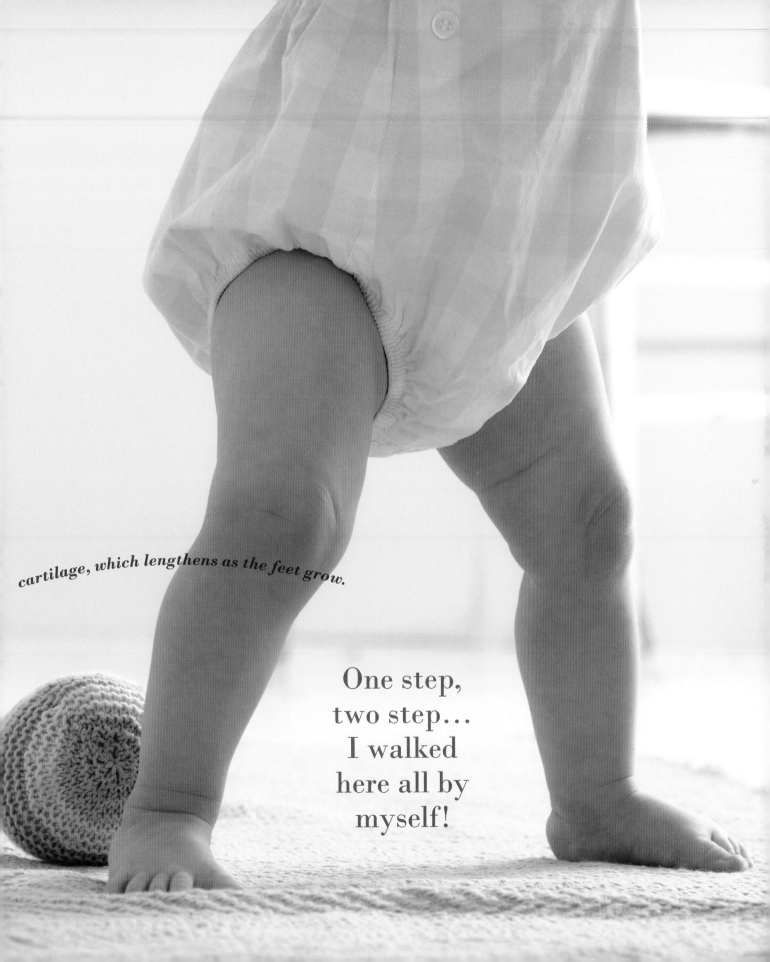

cartilage, which lengthens as the feet grow.

One step,
two step…
I walked
here all by
myself!

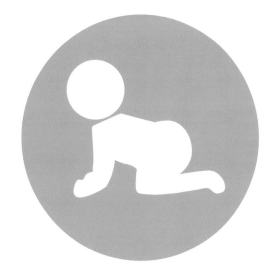

Hello, *gorgeous!*

sleep

* 11–12 hours of sleep at night.
* Usually two daytime naps of about 60 to 90 minutes each.

food

* Eats family food, but often likes things mashed or cut up.
* Can be weaned from breast milk or formula onto cow's milk.

teeth

* Gums may become swollen and uncomfortable as first-year molars start to push through.

"mama, dada"

* Tries to imitate familiar words.
* Has a few words of her own, such as "dada", "mama", "uh-oh", and, very commonly, "milk"!
* Understands simple instructions.

on the move

* Crawls confidently (although some skip this stage or shuffle).
* Pulls up to standing and may cruise around the furniture.
* May stand alone, and even take first independent steps.

I can...

* Wave goodbye.
* Pick things up with a pincer grasp and may be able to hold a chunky crayon.
* Play patty-cake and peekaboo. Understand "no," but may not obey!

my world

* Loves to play outside and will stop to look at everything.
* Is more independent—may not appreciate play being interrupted at bed- or bath-time.
* Plays happily alongside her peers, although doesn't actually interact with them.

I am 12 months old

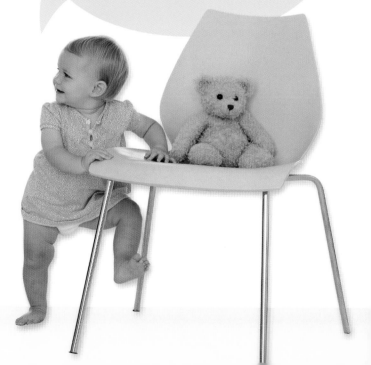

Look at me!
I'm mobile now, and chatter a lot. It won't be long before I take my first steps!

Your little one is finding new ways to express herself. Her increased dexterity means that play gets messier as she grapples with paints and chunky crayons, and noisier as she finds her voice!

Books will engage your toddler completely now as she absorbs the colors, stories, numbers, shapes, faces, and animals, and interacts by touching, pointing, and lifting flaps.

I get it! Her fine motor control and problem-solving ability are developing at a quick pace. A first chunky puzzle with raised handles or knobs is the perfect challenge now.

Your baby adds more words to her repertoire. She understands even more and is noticing the rhythm of speech and conversations.

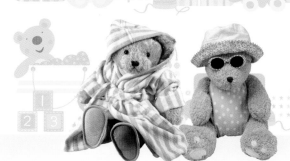

One today

Your baby's first birthday is a wonderful milestone and a time for celebration. It's your first anniversary as his parents, too, so congratulate yourselves!

Planning a party

Your baby's birthday might be the first time you have officially celebrated his arrival. So this may be a chance to get everyone together and share the happy day, or just have a small gathering with close family. Consider your guest list—there may be some "must-have" adults who have children of their own. Can you fit everyone in your home, or do you need a venue? Timing is also important. Make the party fit your baby's routine, so that he enjoys himself and is at his best.

Invitations

It's nice to make the party an occasion by sending out invitations. Store-bought invites are widely available, offering simple designs, or glittery glamour, or children's characters. If you want to get creative, designing your own invitations is easy with websites providing simple design packages. You could include a photo of your baby. Or hand-make invites with blank cards, crafty bits, and photos. Remember to keep one invite as a memento.

Party food

First birthday parties are likely to cater to adults and children alike, and the easiest way to accommodate them all is with basic party food. Sandwiches, pigs-in-a-blanket, and cookies are simply and cheaply provided and are a treat for all age groups. Remember to include snacks for little babies, such as rice cakes, bread sticks, and hummus. A cake is the centerpiece and a key part of the birthday ritual, even if your baby doesn't eat much of it.

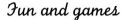

Fun and games

One-year-olds don't need professional entertainers—just putting out some of their favorite toys, including push toys, foam mats, tunnels, blocks, and balls, will be more than enough to keep them entertained. Bubbles are also a real treat and a basic bubble machine causes great excitement. Find a soundtrack of nursery rhymes to play during the party.

If you have a wider age range coming, then you may need to provide something more age appropriate, or at least have room outside for them to run around. A tent in the backyard with a supervising adult might help keep children occupied: some young children will find a large gathering of adults overwhelming so a slightly separated play zone might work well.

At this age you don't need to provide party favors—most traditional contents, such as candy and small plastic toys, are not appropriate anyway. A box of raisins or a tube of bubbles will be an exciting and cheaper alternative. Or, if you really want to go-for-broke, a small soft toy or a board book work well.

Making a birthday memorable

A birthday party can be hectic, but remember when it is over you will long for photographic reminders. Record your baby's special day with lots of photos and videos. You might be running around at crucial moments, so perhaps enlist the help of a family member, and make sure you're in some of the pictures, too. Ask guests to take photos and to email them to you afterward; they will be less busy and might capture more unusual moments.

Before your guests arrive, try to figure out if anything in your home is likely to make the day run less smoothly. Put special toys and breakable objects out of reach, and use stair gates or barricades to cordon off areas where you don't want children to go. Provide a separate diaper-changing area where people can take their babies without having to keep asking.

In many ways, a first birthday party is for you as parents to celebrate your baby, since he won't really remember it. However, you can establish traditions at a first birthday that can then be marked each year. For example, you could make notches on a wall or height chart to record how your child grows each birthday; or take a photograph each year to show how your child is growing and changing. One day he will be able to look back at them all as a sequence of his life.

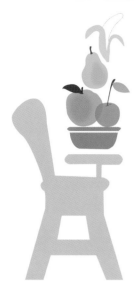

Look what I can *eat!*

Are you obsessed with fruit and vegetables? While your toddler might not be aware of the importance of healthy eating, you can create a broccoli-loving toddler while he is busy tooling up with a fork and spoon and feeding himself.

Your toddler's sense of identity as a separate person from you grows from around 12 months, sparking his mission for more independence. Learning to successfully feed himself is a huge milestone and a crucial part of his social and emotional development. Nurture healthy eating habits now and he'll have a positive attitude toward food for life.

Food power play

Becoming more independent means he wants more control and that includes over his food, so it's no surprise that mealtimes can sometimes feel like a battlefield. Most toddlers go through a phase of being fussy eaters, when they refuse to eat all but a few select foods. Try to avoid the trap of only giving him food you know he'll eat since you'll make it harder to branch out in the long run. Keep offering him simple choices and make positive comments about them. Stay calm and don't turn it into a power struggle.

Rainbow selection

Always offer a wide variety of foods in an array of different colors and textures, and let him see you enjoying them, too. Toddlers are suspicious of new foods so don't expect him to embrace an unfamiliar offering with an open mouth. Perhaps place the new food next to something he already likes to whet his appetite. Keep portions small and don't make it a drama if he refuses to eat something.

Fingers first

Your toddler's hand–eye coordination is maturing every day, and he will gradually gain proficiency at feeding himself with a spoon or fork. But best of all are finger foods—he will love having control over what goes in his mouth, and will enjoy squishing foods between his fingers. Pop a splash mat under his chair and a bib around his neck—and possibly yours, too—since it'll be a messy affair.

> It may take up to ten times of being presented with a new food for your toddler to accept it into his food "repertoire."

"Me do it!"

At about 12–14 months, he'll start trying to feed himself with a spoon, although it may take several months of practice for him to accurately navigate the food into his mouth. Try taking turns, until he masters it. Most toddlers will be confident using cutlery by about 18 months. And this new skill will also boost his self-esteem.

Happy families

Eating together encourages the idea that meals are an opportunity to spend time as a family, and it switches the focus from your toddler to a relaxed, social environment where he may (briefly!) forget to be difficult. Learning the importance of communal eating is an important social skill.

No food is forbidden

To encourage a positive attitude toward healthy eating, avoid labeling foods as "good" or "bad." By completely banning unhealthy foods, such as chocolate or chips, your child will covet them all the more. This doesn't mean that you need to make them a regular part of his diet. Instead opt for a "nothing is forbidden" approach and include these foods as special treats. He'll soon learn that they're not everyday items and will be thrilled when they land on his plate.

Top tips to create a fruit and veggie afficionado

● Whip up a vitamin-packed pasta sauce containing puréed vegetables, such as tomatoes, broccoli, carrots, and peppers. He'll love the taste and as he gets older and more used to it you can leave the vegetables lumpier.

● Finger foods are big winners for toddlers, so offer up some hummus with dipping sticks made out of red pepper or cucumber.

● Make a fun vegetable face—cucumber slice eyes, a tomato nose, red pepper mouth, and romaine heart. Which part will he eat first?

● Pop chunks of fresh fruit into juice when freezing ice pops, or add chunks to Jell-O before it sets in the refrigerator.

Bright young things

A toddler's brain is akin to a hyperactive sponge, soaking up all it can from the world to get ready for the future.

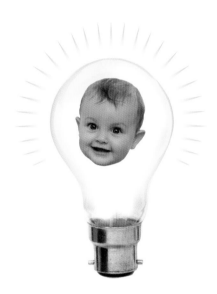

You only have to watch a toddler mastering the use of an iPad in less time than the average adult to realize that they have a staggering capacity to absorb information and learn new skills. This is because their brains have **nearly twice as many synapses**, or connections, and are designed to be highly flexible, allowing new pathways to be created constantly. A newborn's brain is only 25 percent developed, and during the first few years it changes and grows rapidly. This is why experiences during this time, when the brain is twice as active, have a profound and lasting effect on its structure, function, and performance.

> A newborn's brain is only a quarter the size of an adult's, but will grow to 80 percent of adult size by three years old.

Over the past 10 years, cognitive science has made great strides in uncovering the mysteries of **brain development** during the first years of life. Scientists have discovered that the parts of the toddler brain that are most active are the same as those operating in an adult while engrossed in a movie. This suggests that **toddlers view the world as we see a movie—** with excitement and enthusiasm, their attention focused on the visual, and with a heightened ability to adapt to new events.

You may at times find yourself frustrated by your toddler's inability to concentrate, but this apparent lack of focus serves an important purpose. Unlike the "spotlight" consciousness of an adult, which focuses on one thing at a time, the **"lantern" consciousness** of a child spreads its light all around, absorbing as many stimuli as possible from the environment. A vast number of neurotransmitters are produced as all this information is processed, which is the reason why a very young child requires a high concentration of anesthesia to be put to sleep for surgery—they are literally more conscious than an adult.

One of the most impressive skills a toddler learns is the ability to communicate. During their first year, babies' brains are fine-tuned to **distinguish the sounds of language**, which is why only a language that is heard during this initial 12 months can be learned to a truly native level. It is vital to talk to your baby even before she can answer you, since while you are talking her brain is forming the connections that will later enable her to understand and create these sounds for herself. She is distinguishing patterns, learning sounds that will be used repeatedly, and even predicting what is likely to come next. It is interesting to note that in languages in which nouns are assigned a gender, such as French and Spanish, the gender is learned automatically by native speakers, as a part of the word itself. This is something that people coming to the language later in life, when their brain lacks the vital plasticity, may struggle to learn.

Bilingualism boosts brain function and has even been linked to an ability to stave off dementia.

These first few years of heightened brain activity are, of course, the best time to learn an **additional language.** When raising a bilingual child, consistency is key: if, say, you are an English speaker and your partner is French, you should each communicate with your baby only in your own language. Once she is between two and three years old she

should be **able to differentiate between the two languages** and use them in the correct context. She may well favor one language over the other, probably the one that is shared between the parents, but you shouldn't give up on speaking the other—your toddler will be absorbing it even if she is initially resistant to using it. It is also important to respect the inherent cultural connections; songs and stories should be shared in both languages, if possible.

Despite the fact that overall language development can often be slower for bilinguals, knowing how to speak two languages is actually **highly beneficial for brain function**. Both these language systems are always active in the child even when only one is being used, so decisions constantly have to be made about which word to use in a particular context, giving the brain a regular workout.

Once a child grows older and graduates into the teenage years, a kind of **"pruning" process** occurs in the brain. Of the many vastly overproduced synapses, those that have proven less useful over the years will literally shrivel away, leaving only those nerve cells and connections that are vital in daily life to strengthen and remain readily available.

There are easy ways to help your child's brain to achieve its full potential. By simply showing love and affection, and offering plenty of positive stimulation, such as conversation and play, you will actually **influence the chemistry** of the developing brain. Children learn through experience, so the best way to help your toddler improve her skills is by reading to her, talking to her, performing routines, exploring, and playing. However, trying to force development in a particular area can do more harm than good. Children learn at their own rates—their brains are highly absorbent and programmed to learn without any particular intervention from an adult. All you need to do is be with them, love them, listen to them, and involve them in your life—and their smart, flexible little brains will take care of the rest.

Kids just wanna have *fun*

Playfulness and a zest for life are definitely infectious, so show your toddler every day how exciting the world is. Don't miss an opportunity to bond and enjoy each other's company by playing together—and active, physical play is also good exercise for you both!

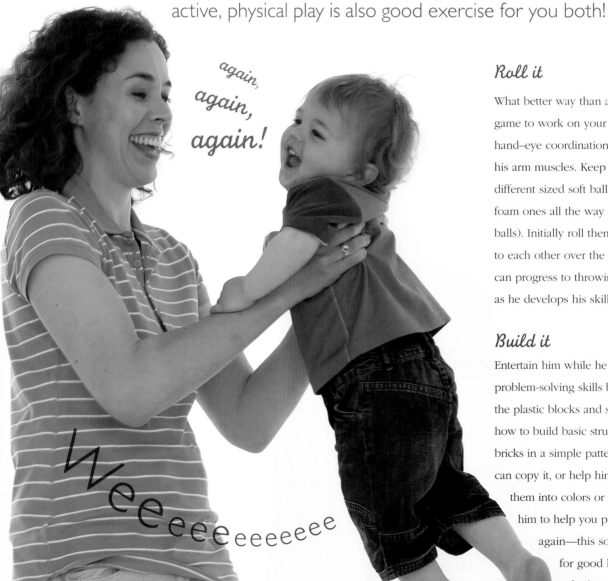

again, again, again!

Weeeeeeeeee

Roll it

What better way than a good ball game to work on your baby's hand–eye coordination and build up his arm muscles. Keep a collection of different sized soft balls (from small foam ones all the way up to beach balls). Initially roll them back and forth to each other over the floor, then you can progress to throwing and catching as he develops his skills.

Build it

Entertain him while he tests out his problem-solving skills by getting out the plastic blocks and showing him how to build basic structures. Put four bricks in a simple pattern and see if he can copy it, or help him to separate them into colors or shapes; then ask him to help you put them all away again—this sows the seeds for good housekeeping for later, too.

Dive right in

Water is fascinating for your little one, and there are lots of ways to enjoy it. Assembling a variety of containers and toys can really spice up bath-time, just as filling a paddling pool can while away a sunny afternoon. Having a little tea party with water, watering the garden together, or giving him a bucket and cloth so he can wash dishes like Mommy will entertain him and train his dexterous fingers.

Get going

He will enjoy any games that test his fledgling walking skills, so moving a sturdy box or a chair for him to hold onto while he takes a few steps will delight him. Similarly, setting up a line of chairs or a selection of supports so he can make it around the room independently will develop his motor skills and build his confidence. Simple obstacle courses with things to crawl under or over will also improve his spatial awareness and balance.

Give him a hand

Clapping games like "Patty-cake," as well as songs with actions like "This Little Piggy" will get your toddler thinking about his hands and figuring out how to use them. Sit opposite him so he can watch you, then switch it around sometimes by having him on your lap, so he can watch your hands from a different perspective and you can guide his into the right positions.

Bring it to life

Bring a favorite toy to life—so Teddy Bear walks around the room on adventures, gets tucked in for naps, and sits at the table for meals. In addition to being fun, this teaches your child about his daily routines, stretches his imagination, and helps him understand emotions, especially if he has to help his bear through sad and happy times. By talking through everything Teddy does you will be exposing your child to lots of useful language, too.

Get out and about

A good walk can be revitalizing and exciting; your little one can either look at the world going by from the stroller, or (if he is already walking) he can hop out and stretch his legs. Take along a ball to play with in the park or a bucket so he can pick up things he is interested in, and test out the swings and the slide. Soft-play centers provide him with lots of ways to build strength and learn new movements, and heading to a local swimming pool for a splash is invigorating and good exercise for you both.

Move it and shake it

Once your little one has found his feet, there are lots of games you can play to develop his new walking abilities. Hide-and-seek is a perennial favorite, since he is chasing and being chased—he'll probably get so excited by these games that he won't even notice he is building up leg strength and improving his balance. Dancing to different types of music will encourage him to adjust his movements to suit the mood, using his imagination and working on his sense of rhythm.

Bolster independence

As much as you love to play with your toddler, it is also important that he learns how to play by himself. Try putting him in a playpen (perhaps in the kitchen while you are cooking) and give him some safe household items that he sees you use, such as plastic spoons, strainers, or pans, to play with. Or get him started on a game with toys then quietly move to a different part of the room and see how long he will continue without your input. Try it again each day, and he will gradually rely on his own imagination for entertainment.

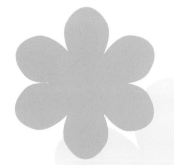

"I'm a snowman!"
From 18 months or
so, toddlers love
games that involve
dressing up and
escaping to
imaginary worlds.

When your toddler discovers that she can do something for herself—be it rolling a ball or using a crayon—she'll be thrilled, and her success will spur her on and make it more likely she'll try out new things.

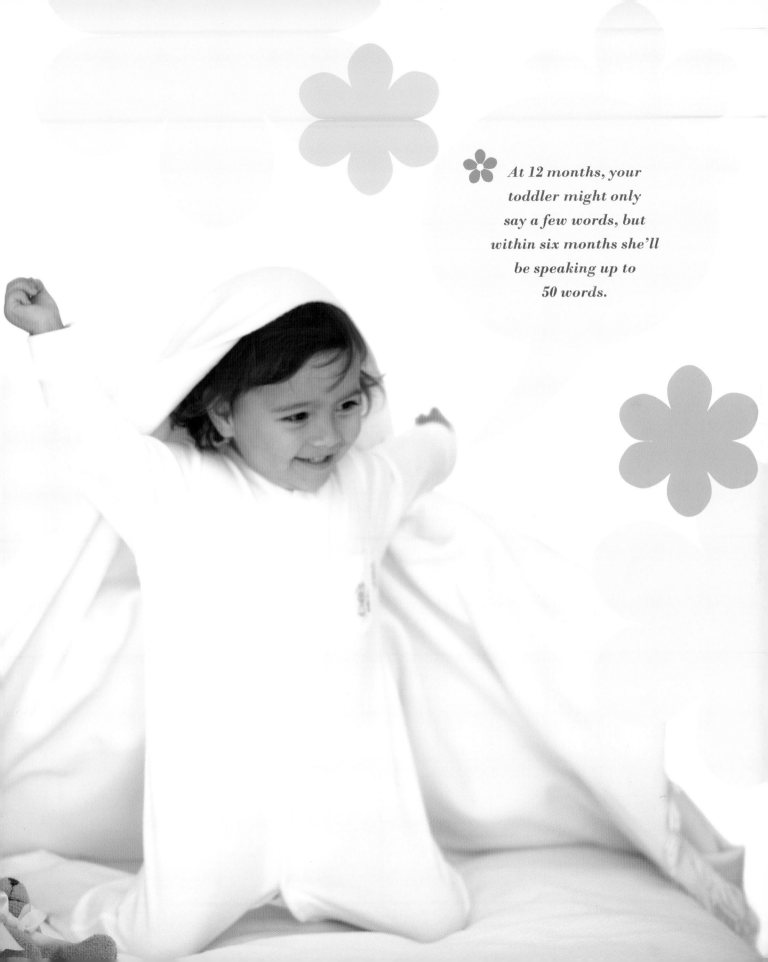

At 12 months, your toddler might only say a few words, but within six months she'll be speaking up to 50 words.

Look what I can do!

Now that your baby is in her second year she is becoming more active and independent. Her personality is blossoming and she's an affectionate, giggly whirlwind of fun.

Clever hands

Your toddler's fine motor skills are now refined enough to pick up objects and put them into a container, stack blocks on top of each other, play with a shape-sorter box, and carefully pick up tiny objects, such as raisins, between finger and thumb in a pincer movement. At around 13 months, she may be able to scribble with crayons. Her hand–eye coordination allows her to point at pictures and turn pages when you read to her.

By playing with her you can actively help develop and improve her dexterity, for example, give her a box of things that are fun to prod, squeeze, and crumple—tissue paper, a roll of tape, and playdough.

Encourage her to empty and fill up a small canvas bag, to push large beads into a small bottle, and to feed large wooden curtain rings over a stick.

Let's get physical

By the time she's one year old, your baby will have usually tripled her birthweight and grown about 10 in (25 cm) taller. Growth slows down between the ages of one and two years, but she's still growing rapidly. She may already be walking—or soon will be—and her world is opening up. She's very physical and will want to clamber over furniture and explore your home. The stairs will be very appealing: she can climb up but might not know how to get back down, and you will need to stay close by. Pulling, pushing, throwing balls, and knocking things down are favorite activities. Help improve her gross motor skills with swimming, dancing, and bouncing on a mini trampoline.

Social skills

Between 12 and 18 months, your toddler's sense of identity strengthens—she'll recognize herself in the mirror instead of thinking it's another child. Usually she'll respond to her own name and refer to herself with it. She becomes more aware of how she fits into your family and, being naturally curious about people, will respond to smiles and attention. Although she'll enjoy being around other toddlers she will probably only play alongside them in parallel play, rather than actually playing with them. At around 18 months, she may start interacting more, but will find the concept of sharing toys hard! Through play, she'll eventually learn how to negotiate and compromise. By 18 months, she can say between 8 and 40 words but will understand far more than she'll yet be able to communicate.

Praise her for saying "please" and "thank you"—pleasing you will encourage her to say them even more.

If you make a rule—such as holding your hand near the street—stick to it. By giving in to tears or a tantrum you will teach her that she can get her own way if she pushes you.

Emotional development

Your toddler is egocentric and views the world solely from her perspective. She's still learning to cope with her own feelings and simply cannot see things from another viewpoint. Separation anxiety—becoming upset when you leave her—is very common (see pages 236–237). She has no concept of time so doesn't know when—or if—you'll be back. But it shows she's forged a strong attachment to you. Make goodbyes easier by keeping them short with a kiss and reassurance—she'll often stop crying the minute you're out of sight. Becoming more independent boosts her self-confidence. Encourage this by letting her wander off from your side in the park to the slide (obviously while keeping a close eye on her!) and see if she will roam around toddler-proofed rooms at home by herself.

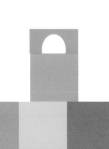

On best behavior

Your toddler learns from you how to behave and act. Children aren't born knowing how to take part in family life and society, so it's up to you to help her join in happily and safely (with just a few tantrums along the way).

Talk to her directly

Use your child's name to get her attention before you ask her to do something, for example, "Daisy, please go get your shoes." Use eye contact so you know she can hear you and that she's listening. For a child under three, it's a good idea to bend or sit down to be at her eye level. Keep your language clear and simple, and ask her to repeat what you said, and if she can't, make it simpler. Try to give one direction at a time so she can process it easily.

Use positive language

If you focus on the negative, for example, "don't drop that plate," she'll focus on an image in her head of dropping the plate. If you say "please give that plate to Mommy" she will focus on doing that. The subconscious brain, even in adults, can't process negatives—which is why if we are told: "don't think of an elephant," that's the first thing we'll think of!

Praise, rather than criticize

Repeatedly telling a toddler that she is "a very naughty girl" or "being a baby" leads to poor self-esteem. Instead, praise what she does well, for example, "I like the way you helped your brother," or "I love it when you help me tidy up." Phrases such as these show her what you do want and boost her confidence, too. However, don't be afraid to use a firm, strong "no" when you need to. Knowing when "no" really means "no" could be

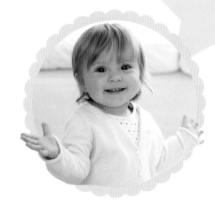

essential one day, if your experimental toddler is about to pick up something sharp or do something dangerous.

Stop the orders

If you are constantly barking orders such as "stop that," "come here," or "go and do this," a child often can't see why they should do what you want. By rephrasing it: "I would like you to come over here please," or "I would like you to stop taking Tom's toy away from him," it takes the focus away from her and onto you, and she will find it easier to change her behavior.

Give a little notice

Children find it hard to switch their attention suddenly when they are absorbed in play, so try giving her a little notice to prepare for the next activity. For example, by saying, "we'll be going in five minutes, start putting away the dolls," or "it's almost time to go, say goodbye to Tom please," you enable her to be ready when you are.

When, not if

Toddlers can't always understand what "if" means. "If you come and brush your teeth, I'll read you a story," doesn't always get results. Using the word "when" is better: "when we've brushed your teeth, we'll read a story," gives your child a clear expectation and tells her you know she will do it as asked.

Give limited choices

Open-ended choices can be a little overwhelming for young children, but a simple choice such as "do you want cereal or toast?" will facilitate an answer, and gives your child some sense of independence.

Use your ps and qs

You are your child's role model. You may think she is too young to notice you saying "please" and "thank you," but it will show her that this is the norm. If you use social niceties, and reinforce them to your toddler, she will copy you—and your friends will be very impressed!

Toddlers are born mimics—keep in mind your own phrases and actions may well enter her repertoire.

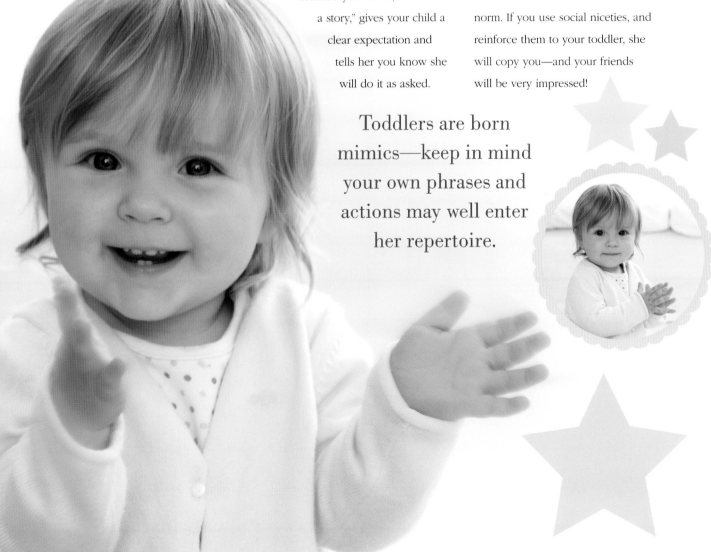

Don't go

Now and then you'll need to leave your baby with someone else—whether it's for an appointment, a night out, or a baby-free shopping trip. Separation anxiety causes these tears and clinginess, but knowing how to handle it can make all the difference.

The panic begins

Once your toddler notices that you are a separate person—and so can leave—he starts to worry that you won't return, which triggers tears and clinginess, commonly known as separation anxiety. It can strike from around eight months and is a normal developmental stage that usually passes by the age of two, though expect recurrences with stressful situations, such as a change of caregiver.

Anxiety triggers

Separation anxiety can be triggered by a fear of new people and/or unfamiliar situations—so while some babies are happy being left with grandma, they may start screaming in a less familiar place, such as a new playgroup. For others, any degree of separation can cause a reaction. It doesn't affect all babies, however: some personalities are naturally ebullient, others more wary. So you may be lucky!

Getting inside his head

It's easiest to act appropriately if you understand what's going on in your baby's head. The words "want Mommy" really mean, "I don't feel safe, I don't trust these people to take care of me, and I don't know if you will ever come back." With experience, he'll learn he can trust you to return, especially as his memory improves. Until then, give lots of reassurance, and try to help him get used to the idea.

Handling the tears

The best course of action is not to stop going out—shackling yourself to your child is not healthy on either side: you need freedom and he needs to learn to cope without you. Start by soothing your toddler's basic anxieties about feeling safe, trusting someone else, and believing you'll come back. Make sure he is comfortable in the new setting and has bonded with the caregiver—and that you feel reassured, too. Explain what's going to happen—he'll understand more than he's able to say.

Walk out the door

To the dreaded leaving, then. Act upbeat even if you feel rotten or guilty, settle him with an activity or a hug from the caregiver, then say goodbye cheerily, and with a kiss. Be upbeat, not nervous—or he will be, too—and, however great the temptation, don't slip away while he's not looking, or (even more tempting) come back immediately. Try not to stand behind the door listening to the screams, just get on your way and call later for reassurance. Finally, return when you promised (or a bit before).

So, now you're back

While your toddler may run toward you for an embrace, or even burst into relieved tears, there is a chance that he won't actually notice or, worse, say "don't want Mommy." Though it may cut like a knife, remember you have taken a positive step toward cracking the tears. Parenting is a long struggle to balance both your needs and your child's need for independence, and when either of you moves toward that goal, the other can feel rejected. Think of it as preparation for parenting a teenager!

Heartbreaking as it can be, each time you leave your child will make it a little easier the next time, and the next, until he is happy to wave goodbye to you.

"Don't leave me here, Mommy."

sleep

* 11–12 hours of sleep at night.
* Usually a one- to two-hour afternoon nap, or two shorter naps.

food

* Eats family food, three times a day, and enjoys regular snacks, using an easy-grip spoon, but not always very accurately.
* Drinks independently from her cup.

teeth

* About 12 teeth, with first-year molars making an appearance.
* Needs helps brushing with a soft brush.

I know that!

* Holds finger to mouth and says "shhh."
* Recognizes names of familiar people, objects, and body parts.
* Points to an object when it's named.
* Has between 8 and 40 recognizable words, maybe more.

on the move

* Squats to pick up a toy.
* Climbs into an armchair, turns, and sits.
* Kicks a big ball, but not very accurately.
* May be able to master a big tricycle.

I can...

* Take off some items of clothing.
* Push and pull toys while walking.
* Sort toys into colors, shapes, and sizes.
* Build towers three or four blocks high.

my world

* More confident and social.
* May exert will and is resisting going to bed— and learning to climb out of it.
* Eager to try things by herself.
* Generally social and very spontaneous.

I am 18 months old

Look at me!
I'm walking, talking, and taking my first real steps towards independence.

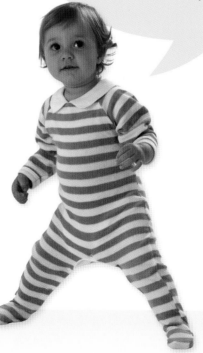

Your 18-month-old will soon become a super-scribbler as her dexterity and attention span grow and her imagination takes off. Encourage her emerging creativity with a case of pencils and crayons.

Your toddler is increasingly social and relaxed with her peers, and may even have a favorite friend. As her social skills improve, she starts to observe and learn the art of sharing!

Your toddler is starting to grasp the two-way conversation, learning to take turns, and using words more to get her meaning across. Your rapt attention encourages her to talk on and on.

 Don't go! Her growing independence makes her a little nervous too, and she's anxious when you leave her. Separation anxiety peaks at this age.

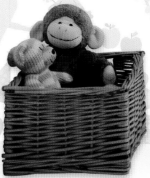
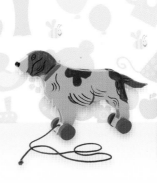

Upwardly *mobile*

By now your toddler will be eager to run around as fast as his little legs can carry him. He also has zero sense of danger so it's a juggling act for you to keep him happy and safe.

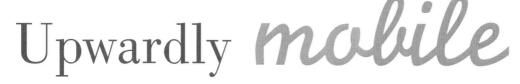

As your toddler grows, you will find yourself constantly having to balance rules with play—setting and enforcing these boundaries is key to his development.

On the move

By 18 months, your toddler is walking well without exaggerated high steps. A few months later, he can also walk backward and sideways and may run, albeit stiffly. By the age of two, he'll be running quite fast, although he may find it difficult to change direction or glance over his shoulder without crashing or falling over.

Hold my hand!

Make your expectations clear when you're setting boundaries. Be specific: don't just say he must be a "good boy," instead say something like: "you must hold my hand when we're walking along the street, it keeps you safe." When he obeys, praise him to reinforce his good behavior, and keep a positive note by talkting to him about what you are planning to do when you reach your destination.

> By explaining your reasons, you will help him to understand why he shouldn't do a particular thing.

Rein him in?

The parenting jury is out on putting toddlers in reins; however, there's no right or wrong—the priority is to keep your child safe. If you need to walk along busy streets, reins might be a good idea, whereas in the park he might be fine: you know your child and his wanderlust best, so trust your judgement.

My little runaway

Why do toddlers run off? Because they can! It's the heady mix of having more independence and the freedom of running. Explain why he shouldn't, and try not to laugh or he'll think it's a game and do it more often.

Give him some freedom

Your toddler's desire to run is natural, so give him that freedom safely. If you can see him in safe, open space, let him run ahead of you. He'll probably turn around to check that you're there, but keep him in sight and stay close. Show him where it's safe to run—in the park, for instance, you don't want him to disappear into the bushes.

The great outdoors

Go outside with your toddler even if it's raining. Playing outside is good for his health and physical confidence so give him the space to run, jump, kick, throw, and use his natural energy. He will love swings and slides, and the occasional falling off something is all part of the learning experience. He loves exploring and learning more about his ever-expanding world—he'll just need rain boots and jacket some days.

Indoor soft play

You probably never set foot in an indoor play area before you became a parent, but they can be great if the weather isn't good. Your toddler has fun and can let off steam in a safe, controlled environment. You'll still have to keep a close eye on him, as, although usually supervised, you're still responsible for his behavior and well-being.

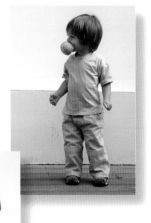

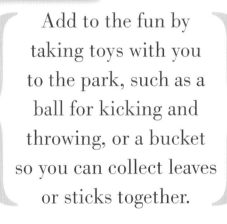

{ Add to the fun by taking toys with you to the park, such as a ball for kicking and throwing, or a bucket so you can collect leaves or sticks together. }

Again, again! Endless repetition

and physical play come into their

own now. So, who's up for

another round of hide and seek?

…Peekboo, Mommy!

Here I come, ready or not!

Between the ages of 18 months and 2 years, curiosity becomes the governing force of your toddler's actions. Toddlers want to explore constantly, whether its peering around a corner to see who's there, or teetering on the edge of the forbidden staircase to see what you say, or even walloping another child on the head to see what happens. Everything is about experimentation—what happens if…

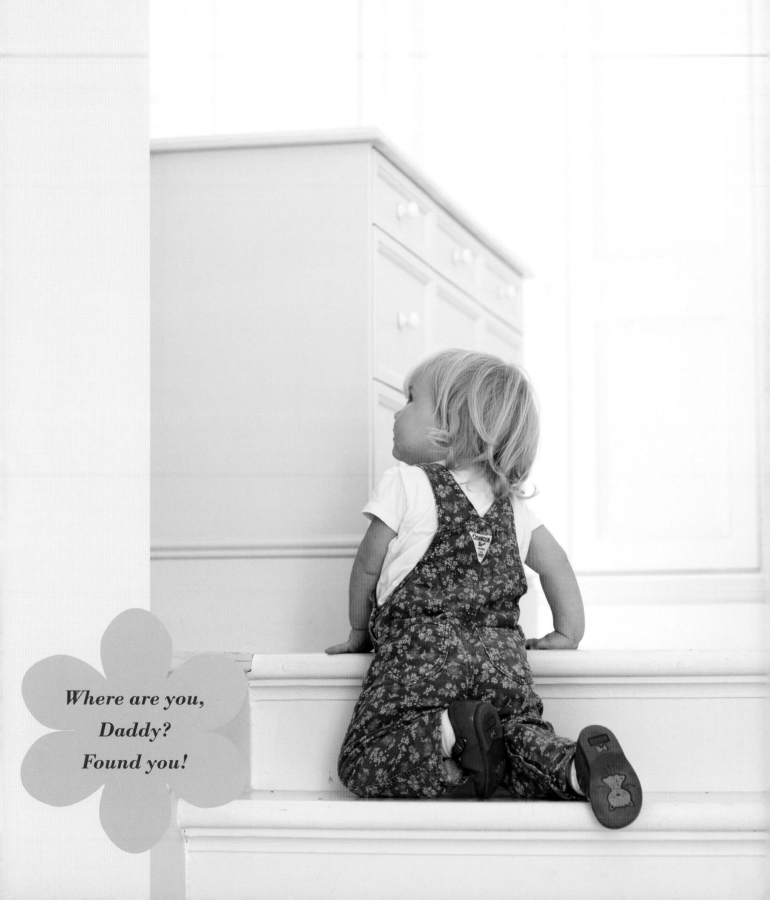

Where are you, Daddy? Found you!

Talk to me

You may feel in need of a translator when your toddler first begins to talk—confusion and misunderstandings can result in tantrums. But there are plenty of things you can do to improve her communication skills.

After months of cooing and babbling followed by increasing word recognition, your toddler is going to be eager to expand her linguistic repertoire. First, though, she has to coordinate dozens of vocal and facial muscles, so it's not surprising her early attempts to speak are muddled. Once she is able to communicate initial things to you, she may become upset when you are then unable to understand the less comprehensible parts of her chatter. For your child to articulate words clearly, the muscles in her face, mouth, and tongue first need to develop, and there are simple ways that you can encourage this.

A study in 2012 showed that babies first learn language

Fun with straws Engaging your toddler in fun, physical activities, such as blowing bubbles through a straw, can help her acquire the more complex mouth movements that are used during speech. In fact, sucking from a straw, particularly from denser textures such as yogurt, is a technique used by speech therapists to develop oral muscles. Introducing a regular smoothie time each week can act as a tasty treat and a facial work out in one—she'll need little encouragement to pick up the straw.

Food for talk Foods that require extra chewing can also help to develop the muscles involved in talking. By punctuating your toddler's day with healthy snacks such as sliced apples and pears, you will encourage her to exercise her jaw in more ways than one!

In my imagination Toddlers who engage in imaginative play can improve their language skills, and around the age of two your toddler is primed to enter the world of make-believe. Encourage her to dress up and create miniature "worlds" and watch as she adapts her language to imaginary situations, helping her make significant cognitive leaps.

 Sing-along Familiarizing your toddler with songs and rhymes from an early age will enhance her listening skills, and help her to identify different sounds and to recreate them. The repetition in nursery rhymes makes the words easier to remember, while the rhythm in music and rhyme echoes the natural rhythms of speech.

Tackle tricky beasts Make up games to help your toddler with her pronunciation of difficult consonants such as "s" and "l." Try linking them with exciting noises, for example "The snake says 'ssssss,'" "The truck says 'bbrrmm bbrrmm.'" The winning combination of interaction with you, stimulating noises, and repetition will engage her and encourage her to tackle some trickier sounds.

 Copy cat After watching and reading your lips while you're creating a sound, your toddler can then try it herself. So, make sure she can see your face when you talk to her.

through watching the shapes your lips make.

 Learn through play Conversational skills can be improved through games that mirror a two-way conversation, such as rolling a ball between you and saying a word each time you catch it. Back and forth adult–child talking has even more effect on language development than one-way activities, such as reading, since actively conversing gives toddlers a forum to practice talking, make mistakes, and be gently corrected.

Words to the wise

Use gestures and facial expressions when talking to her, as it enriches your communication and reassures her that there's more than one way to get a message across. **Give her time** since it can often take her a little while to find the right word. Resisting the temptation to jump in will boost her confidence, since she'll feel she has time to express herself. **Be careful not to overcorrect her—** a sure-fire way to dampen her enthusiasm— but do gently correct persistent mistakes.

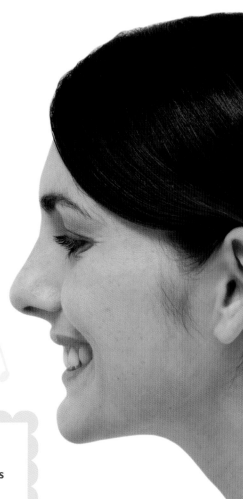

Food
on the go

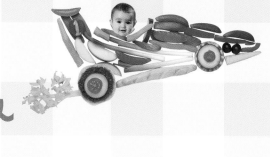

While three nutritious meals a day are essential for growing minds and bodies, snacks are another staple on any toddler's daily menu. Choose foods that are high in energy but packed with goodness to keep blood sugar levels stable and avoid fatigue-induced tantrums.

Hummus

This puréed chickpea dip has a nutty flavor, is thick enough not to be too messy, and is full of folates, vitamin B6, and iron. Children love dipping cut-up vegetables or pita bread in.

DIY mixtures

Make your own version—toss together a combination of low-salt pretzels, whole-grain cereal, goldfish crackers, shaved coconut, chocolate chips… whatever inspires you. Avoid nuts because they can be a choking hazard for children under age 3. This snack is best suited to older toddlers who can chew thoroughly.

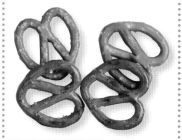

Dried fruit

Raisins contain fiber, potassium, and lots of vitamins, but be creative and expand your repertoire to include dried apples, apricots, and cranberries, too. They taste sweet and children love them. For younger toddlers, you may need to soften them by soaking beforehand.

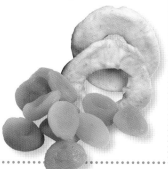

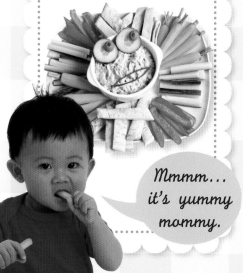

Mmmm… it's yummy mommy.

Cheese

The protein in this child-friendly snack keeps energy levels high. Simple cubes in a plastic cup are easy to carry around, or rustle up some cheese cube "kebabs" at home by alternating with some fruit.

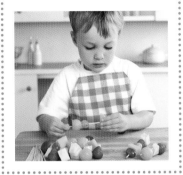

Secret muffins

If you have time for a bit of baking, try out recipes using fruit and vegetables—bananas, zucchini, sweet potatoes, or carrots, for instance. These high-fiber versions are portable parcels of nutritiousness so are perfect healthy treats.

DID YOU KNOW?

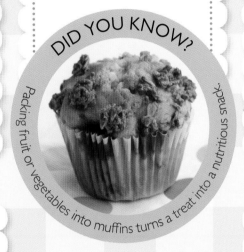

Packing fruit or vegetables into muffins turns a treat into a nutritious snack.

Crispbreads, crackers, and rusks

Opt for versions with no added sugar, and very little salt (sodium). Anything with more than 500 mg per per 3½ oz (100 g) is too salty for young children. Some baby varieties are packaged into handy sizes, which can be stowed for emergencies out of sight in your handbag.

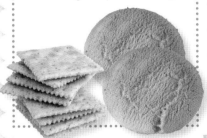

Vegetable chips

Make your own vegetable chips and bag them up to take out with you. Whatever vegetable you choose—sweet potato, parsnip, carrot, and beet all work well—simply slice thinly and bake in the oven with a healthy fat.

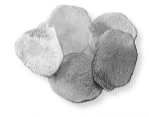

Yogurt

All young bones need calcium, and yogurt has it in bucket loads. Portable bought pouches and tubes are great if you're out, and dress it up at home with berries and granola.

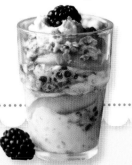

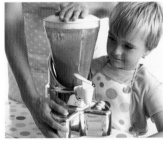

Smoothies

Whether they help pop in the fruit or just press the button, toddlers love smoothies. Improvise with what's in the fridge and fruit bowl; they are great portable frozen treats.

Hair-raising matters

Some babies are born with a full head of hair, others are bald for months. And when is it time for a trip to the salon?

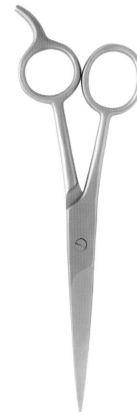

While your baby's hair is probably something she has only ever considered fleetingly—something to tug or tangle—it may be important to you. After all, hair, hairstyles, and hairy issues often preoccupy us as adults, and it seems our children's hair—or lack of it—is a big issue for us, too. Are they born bald or hairy? Will the hair fall out? Will it change color? And when it does grow, who will cut it?

First, whether your child is born with **a smooth pate or a luxuriant mane** comes down to genetics. And whatever amount of hair she does or doesn't have when she emerges into the world, it is likely to change fairly quickly anyway. Babies who are born with hair often lose it during the first six months of life. This is because **hair growth has different phases**. Hair that begins its growth phase in utero will eventually enter a resting (nongrowth) phase and begin to fall out—although not always completely. Hair loss is also partly caused by a hormonal shift within the baby—during pregnancy, your hormones **pass across the placenta** to your baby, and although these hormones remain temporarily present in her body at birth, their levels naturally start to decline shortly afterward, resulting in hair loss.

The speed at which regrowth occurs varies, and when the hair does grow back it may be a **different color or texture**. Some babies can remain bald until after they are a year old—although they often have fine, silky down covering their scalp. Once a baby's hair starts to grow properly,

In some cultures, parents shave a newborn's head, in others they wait until a child can speak before cutting his hair for the first time.

though, parents then have to decide **how to manage it**. Generally speaking this is purely a parental concern, yet in some countries early hair management follows the dictates of age-old customs. All around the world, people have different **hair etiquette**. A Chinese baby, for instance, receives a first haircut at a month old—the head is shaved leaving just a tuft at the crown, and parents then keep the cut hair. Hindus believe any hair from birth is impure and associated with maternal dependence, so the child is shaved in a ceremony known as Chudakarana, which signifies cleansing. Traditional Jewish families do not cut a boy's hair until his third birthday, when he is considered ready to embark on education—this milestone is marked with a formal **haircutting ceremony**. In an ancient Japanese tradition, the lock from a baby's first haircut is preserved and turned into a calligraphy brush—this is believed to secure good fortune for the child. Some parents in the US and the UK also save a lock of baby hair as a memento. Usually, though, the timing of this trim has more to do with practicalities than ritual—the length of the child's hair (can she see where she is going?), her ability to support her own head, and her tolerance for sitting (relatively) still.

So, when the time comes, do you do it yourself or head to the professionals? The advantage of DIY is that it's free and your baby will be more at ease. The downside is that you are susceptible to the effects of your own shaking hand! If nerves prove problematic, you could try cutting your toddler's hair while she's asleep. Either way, **use sharp scissors**—you may think blunt ones will be safer, but they'll pull at the hair and result in an uneven cut.

If you choose to go to a hairdresser's, remember it will be full of sights, noises, and textures that are unfamiliar and possibly frightening to a toddler. Try to **ease the experience** by taking her to watch you get a haircut, or if this is not practical play "hairdressers" with her at home. Some child-

The timing of a baby's first haircut often coincides with a classic stage of wariness of strangers, which can make a trip to the barber tricky...

friendly salons even do a "first haircut" package, which includes a photo and certificate as part of the deal. Get the hairdresser to swing the chair away from the mirror if seeing the scissors bothers her. Or let her sit on your lap.

After a few years, a child's hair thickens and can start to change color. African hair often changes from soft to more wiry at this stage, and children born with blond, strawberry-blond, light-brown, or red hair might find it darkens as they grow. Certain genes responsible for hair color can be turned on or off during early childhood and puberty, and as children grow their levels of the **pigment melanin increase,** which also makes hair naturally darker.

Whatever your child's hair type, she will inevitably end up with that bane of childhood bath-times—**tangled hair**. Children have sensitive scalps, and combing out tangles can be painful. You can buy detangling sprays, but you can make your own, too: just mix one part of your own conditioner with three parts of water in a spray bottle, and lightly spray your child's towel-dried hair before combing using a wide-toothed comb. For true tangle emergencies—involving "foreign bodies" such as sticky candy or dried paint—wet the hair a little and apply baby oil, or even olive oil. Work it in with your fingers and comb through.

Eventually, regular haircuts will become a routine part of your child's life, together with the inevitable disasters, such as your child cutting off a chunk of those angelic locks. Just remember hair will always grow back.

Thinking *big*

sleep

* 10–12 hours of sleep at night. May wake at night, even if she slept well before.
* One daytime nap of one to three hours.
* May be ready for a big bed with a raised side.

food

* May be constantly hungry, but needs small portions since her tummy isn't big enough to hold much food.
* Family meals and healthy, nutritious snacks are important to keep her going.

teeth

* Second-year molars appear between 22 and 30 months, and may be painful.

listen to me!

* Asks for things by name.
* Can put together simple phrases ("more juice") and two-word sentences, ("bye-bye, Mommy").
* Uses pronouns, such as "mine."
* Speaks at least 50 words, and understands many more.

on the move

* Jumps with both feet and stands on tiptoes.
* Walks downstairs alone and up with help.
* Runs avoiding obstacles, and climbs onto furniture and small jungle gyms.

I can...

* Wash and dry hands with help.
* Draw lines, circles, and dots.
* Put on some items of clothing but might not always want to.

my world

* Is determined and curious.
* Understands more about time, including "sooner" and "later."
* Appreciates rewards for positive actions.

I am 2 years old

Look at me!
I'm talkative, curious, and often determined, and my enthusiasm for life is infectious!

Your toddler is great company: full of energy and up for a laugh. She looks to you as a sounding board, there to share her fun and answer repeated questions. When you confirm information, she feels secure.

Balance, coordination, and agility are improving, and outdoor activities come into their own. She's on-the-go: eager to climb, bounce, run, and kick a ball.

Your child's imagination starts to soar. Role play and make-believe begin to take center stage now as she discovers the delights of dressing up, imaginary worlds, and teddy bear picnics!

Her confidence is growing in line with her abilities. Security, routines, and reassurance all help her feel safe enough to "let go."

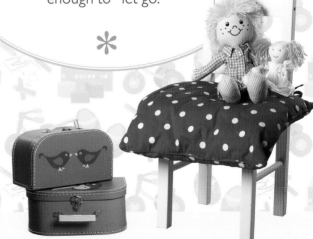

Healthy eating habits for life

Food is one of life's great pleasures, and sharing good food with your child can be a real adventure—exciting but also a little turbulent. We are lucky that most countries have an enormous variety of delicious, healthy, and affordable foods to choose from. So, here's to a lifetime of family favorites mixed in with a few new things along the way.

How much does your toddler need?

A toddler's appetite varies enormously: some days he may eat a lot, especially if he is going through a growth spurt or has had a very active few days; other days hardly at all. If he's drinking lots of water and has the energy to run around, he's fine.

On the menu

According to the US Department of Agriculture, children between the age of two and five need a varied menu, with foods from each food group every day. This includes two small servings of meat, fish, or legumes; four servings of low-fat dairy foods; five servings of fruit and vegetables; and four servings of grains (including breads and cereal).

Little and often

Your toddler has a small stomach, about the size of one of his closed hands, so he needs to eat little and often. Toddlers are good at listening to their bodies, and if he says he is full, he probably is. He will need snacks between meals, and these form an essential part of his diet so have some healthy options available such as fruit, cheese, or vegetable sticks.

Your little helper

Show your child that food is a natural part of everyday life. Help him grow some vegetables, and choose fruit at the market. Encourage him to suggest his favorite meals and prepare them together. He could help you mix a cake, make a sandwich, or put cut-up fruit in a bowl.

Doing it all himself

Your toddler will love to do things himself as it asserts his independence. He will want to feed himself as much as possible, so provide easy-grip spoons and lots of finger foods.

Use your imagination

Toddlers are visual creatures and appetite is stimulated by what they see, so make your child's food look varied and delicious. Offer a selection of foods that display a rainbow of colors, such as ripe tomatoes, carrots, green beans, and cheese, as well as a variety of different textures, including soft, crunchy, and chewy to keep him interested. There's no need to make faces or shapes with food, but funky plates, straws, and lunch boxes will help make it look appealing.

A mini food critic

As adults, there are plenty of foods we don't like much, for example under-ripe tomatoes, processed cheese, soggy vegetables, or bland flavors. Similarly, your child will have his own likes and dislikes, and to an extent these should be accommodated (although check first that he's not just being fussy!). He may also like foods that you don't like yourself, so give him the chance to try new things that aren't on your normal register.

Trying something new

Toddlers can go through phases of trying new things, and other times be fussy and reject old favorites. They like the familiar and may need to be offered a new food as many as 10 times before they eat it.

Dessert bribery

Tempting as it is, try not to tell your child that he can't have dessert if he hasn't finished his main course because it sets up the dessert as the reward.

Make dessert nutritious in its own right, for example yogurt or fruit, and include it as a normal part of any mealtime.

Keeping it short

A restless toddler will be ready to go as soon as he has finished eating, so keep mealtimes fairly short, no longer than 20 minutes or so.

Eating together

Try to share mealtimes and snacks as often as possible: go on a picnic in the yard, enjoy a beverage together in a café, and eat meals at home together. Seeing you eat a range of foods will encourage your child to try new things and will help him to see meals as a social, family occasion.

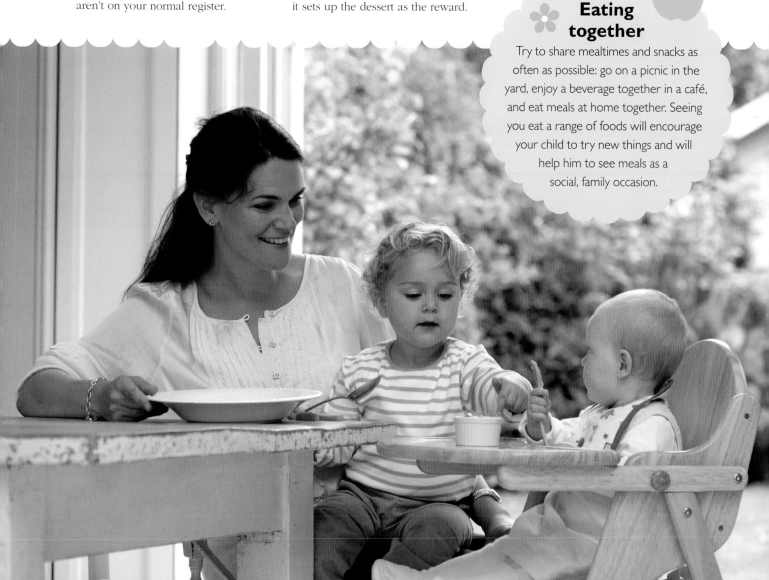

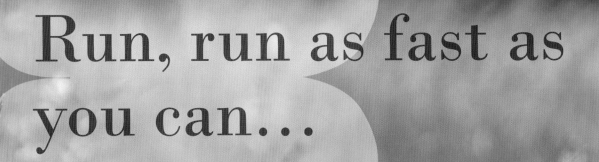

Run, run as fast as
you can...

Enjoy being
outside with
your child—it
benefits you
both.

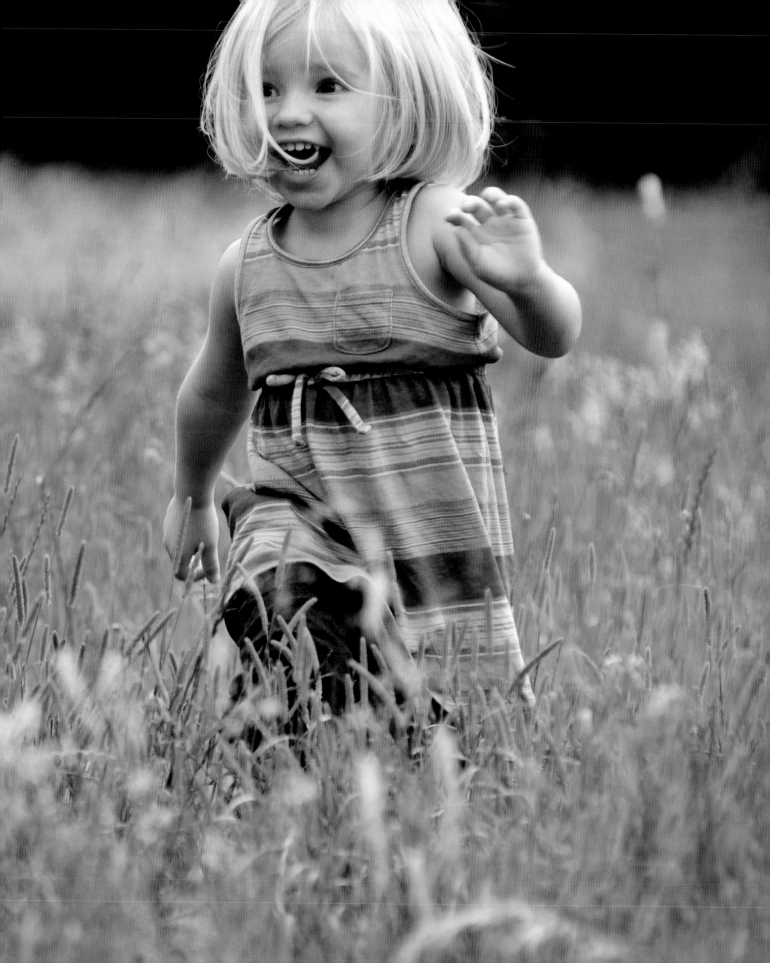

Little *chef*

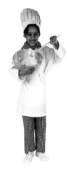

Teaching children to cook gives them life-long skills and fosters a healthy attitude to food. It's never too early to start: all kids enjoy "helping" Mom or Dad, and cooking together can be great fun.

Cooking doesn't get tougher than this!

There's no getting around it—cooking with toddlers is messy! Flour will cover every surface, and the kitchen floor will need to be mopped afterward. Your toddler also works slowly and often just wants to fast forward to licking out the bowl. So don't cook with her if you're feeling tired or time is limited, since you need plenty of patience to make it an enjoyable experience.

Healthy choices

Since child obesity is on the rise in many countries it's vital to help your toddler learn about nutrition and healthy eating right from the start. Growing up with fast food available everywhere, she needs you to equip her with the knowledge to make informed food choices and be able to cook using fresh, nutritious ingredients.

Food lab

You're not just giving your child a cooking lesson; you're teaching her counting, measuring, new vocabulary, and science. She's also practicing her fine motor skills, precision, hand–eye coordination, and artistic skills. Let her spoon mixture into muffin containers and thread fruit onto skewers; her attempts will get better each time.

Encourage experiments

Involving your little chef in choosing, preparing, and helping to cook food, will make her more likely to try new foods. Take her shopping and let her see meat, fruit, and vegetables before you make casseroles or smoothies. Try free samples from the deli counter with her. Grow your own fruit, herbs, and vegetables in the yard or on a windowsill so she can watch them grow and help you pick them.

We are family

Cooking for your family is nurturing and shows your love, and your child can be part of that, too. Getting her on board makes her feel like she's contributing to family life, and she will thrive on the precious one-on-one time with you.

One spoon for the bowl, two spoons for me...

Let's get cooking

Get busy in the kitchen with your eager cook—there's already a lot she can do:

sift flour

break eggs

mixing

rubbing together

Let your child cut up soft fruits such as banana and raspberries then mix them into yogurt. It will make a nice change from pre-flavored yogurts.

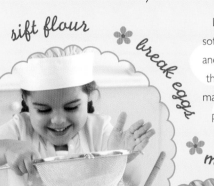

Encourage her to break eggs, sift flour, mix cakes, and try out her decorating skills.

Rubbing butter and flour together for a crumble top is easy and absorbing work for small hands.

kneading dough

cutting pastry

rolling out pasta

Her playdough expertise will make her comfortable kneading dough, rolling out pasta, and cutting out cookie and sandwich shapes.

Recipes

Berry smoothie

Your child can help chop the fruit, and mix all the ingredients together.

Ingredients (serves 4)
5 oz (140 g) hulled strawberries
2 oz (60 g) blueberries or
blackberries
2 peeled bananas
4 fl oz (110 ml) orange juice
13 fl oz (370 g) low-fat plain yogurt

Ask her to chop the fruit using a plastic knife. She can then add all the ingredients to a large bowl and mix everything together.

You put everything into a blender and she can press the button to purée until smooth.

Your sous chef can finish it off by adding a straw to every glass and adding a few extra pieces of fruit.

Chocolate crispy cakes

Enthusiastic kids can measure out the cereal, mix the ingredients, and spoon the mixture into paper cups.

Ingredients (makes 12 cakes)
8 oz (225 g) chocolate
4 oz (125 g) crisped rice or other cereal
2 oz (50 g) raisins or dried apricots

Ask your child to break up the chocolate into chunks and put it into a small glass bowl.

You place the bowl over a saucepan of simmering water, and stir the chocolate until melted.

Pour the chocolate over the cereal, and let your child mix it all together with the fruit. Take it in turns to spoon the mixture into paper cups, let cool, then put in the fridge to set.

What's so terrible about *two?*

It's one of the most overused phrases when referring to this age group, but are the "terrible twos" really so bad?

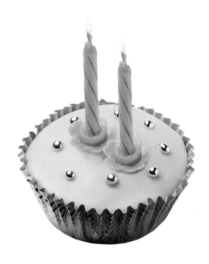

While life with a toddler certainly isn't dull, the very trait that leads to challenging behavior in the first place—a stubborn **quest for independence**—is also what makes your child enthusiastic, lively, funny, and affectionate.

The transition from baby to toddler is one of the most significant developmental leaps that humans experience, so it's not surprising that it's pretty intense, and a tad rocky at times. Your toddler's emotions are raw and immediate, and a **lack of self-consciousness** means that whatever he is feeling is on display for all the world to see—whether at a playgroup, at stores, or at home. The immediacy and strength of his emotions can be stressful to experience, but these are the same feelings that can bowl you over as he flings his arms around you in an enthusiastic embrace. By **maintaining a positive mindset** and making an effort to understand what your child is experiencing, you can make all the difference to family life.

As your child approaches his second year, three significant changes are underway: a growing sense of **self-awareness; increased mobility;** and the **acquisition of language**. A toddler's brain is twice as active as an adult's—no wonder they get tired. The same curiosity that can lead to conflict is also an indication of a healthy interest in the world, and a signal to you that he's ready to interact with more complex stimuli, such as puzzles, challenging toys, varied physical play, and other children and adults. Your child finds the world fascinating, and it's up to you to provide him with the scope to explore it safely and expressively.

At the same time, your child is also developing a growing sense of "me" and will want to let you know his **likes and dislikes**. His vocabulary is growing, almost daily, which means he can express himself more clearly, but this can be challenging for him (and you) since words may not always be clear.

His bid for independence can lead to clashes, but also shows that your child is engaged, active, and learning to deal with life.

He may become rapidly frustrated when you are unable to understand him. Try to think of it as an entertaining and interesting time, as your child learns to interact socially.

All of these developments have a flip side, and this is where toddlers get bad press. As your child's independence grows, he senses that he is increasingly separate from you. So while he is striving to **exert his will**, stepping out on his own can be scary. Add to this frustration the fact that he finds he is not quite able to achieve, or allowed to do, everything he wants, or to communicate his needs effectively, and you have a cocktail of emotions that can lead to a meltdown.

Understanding your **toddler's emotions** is key, and can help you feel more sympathetic. In the journal *Psychology Today*, child psychoanalyst Paul Holinger talks about "translating" your toddler's words into emotions so you understand what he is really trying to communicate. By the age of two, a toddler's emotions are complex, but he only has a limited vocabulary and emotional intelligence. Help him recognize his emotions, so if your toddler tells you to "go away," look at what else is going on. He may actually want you to be closer, and is frustrated that you are not helping. You could say: "I think you are upset with me because I was busy. Would you like me to play?" This gives your child the **words to express himself next time**.

So, what to do if your toddler has a **complete tantrum**? At the peak of a tantrum, your toddler is expressing extreme anger. Researchers at the University of Minnesota discovered a vocal rhythm to tantrums, with certain emotions having their own acoustic features. Peaks of yelling and screaming represented anger, while fussing, whining, and crying shared a similar acoustic group and indicated growing sadness. If you try to intervene at the peak of a tantrum, it could intensify and prolong the episode. So, **take a few deep breaths, and stay calm** and wait until your child calms down, too. He will see that you can cope with his strong emotions and that he can learn to, also.

Avoiding conflict in the first place will help make life easier. A study published in 2012 revealed that when parents consistently responded positively to a toddler's needs, their child developed more **positive attention-seeking behavior**, collaborated more readily, and acted up less. Avoid outings, especially boring ones, when he is tired or hungry. If you notice he is starting to look bored, or like he might misbehave, distract him with a toy he hasn't seen recently.

Toddlers are amazingly fickle: many tantrums can be averted with a quick distraction.

If you want him to sit still at an appointment, take him for a run around outside beforehand. Make life a bit more grown up by giving him simple choices, such as "red socks or blue socks today?" This feeds his need for independence. Praise good behavior when you see it, so your child knows how he is expected to act in a situation, and respond to his requests and questions, even if they are very repetitive.

This is a **fantastic time** to help your child develop into an independent, curious person. Show him how to pace himself, express his needs, and explore the world. Be there to step in and help with new challenges and recognize when it is all a bit overwhelming. This will give him the confidence to take on whatever life presents, and you can watch his own unique personality emerging.

Fun in the *big* outdoors

A desire to explore the big wide world comes naturally to children. And it doesn't matter what the weather is like: children are just as happy making sandcastles in the rain.

Notice the seasons

Head out into the backyard, local park, beach, or woods any time of the year so your child can learn about nature's yearly cycle. Collect fall leaves, pine cones, horse chestnuts, and seedpods to make a home for mini beasts, or take them home to make a collage. Pick flowers and fruit and make piles of grass in the spring and summer. Take a sturdy plastic magnifying glass to add to the sense of discovery.

A world of mini beasts

Become explorers and go on an expedition looking for spiders, beetles, and bugs under rocks, logs, and leaves. Look around you to spot butterflies and birds. How many squirrels can you count? Can you hear any birds, or dogs barking?

Gardening jobs

Whether digging in the garden, watering plants, filling up a bird feeder, or collecting eggs, involve your child in your outdoor jobs (just as you would around the house). It might be routine to you, but it will feel interesting to him, and will build his familiarity with how things grow. Being a helpful part of family life also helps to build his self-confidence and develop a sense of responsibility.

Join the hunt

Plan a mini treasure hunt in a local woods, park, or field. Hide a few small inexpensive toys, notes, or pictures, and encourage your child to look under leaves, behind rocks, and up in low branches. This helps to expand his vocabulary and take in more of his surroundings.

Take a picnic

Eating outdoors is great for the appetite: it might be the fresh air or just simply being somewhere new but everyday food looks a little more appealing when packaged and presented in picnic form. A picnic on the lawn on a sunny day can feel a million miles away; all you need is a blanket and a few sandwiches.

Dip your toes

Children of all ages love water play so take your child for a splash in the puddles, or a paddle in a stream, or find a splash park. If you live near a beach, or are on vacation, walk along the shoreline of a beach and explore rockpools; will you see a fish? Embrace the rain and go outside to get your hair wet, or build a shelter together to escape from the rain.

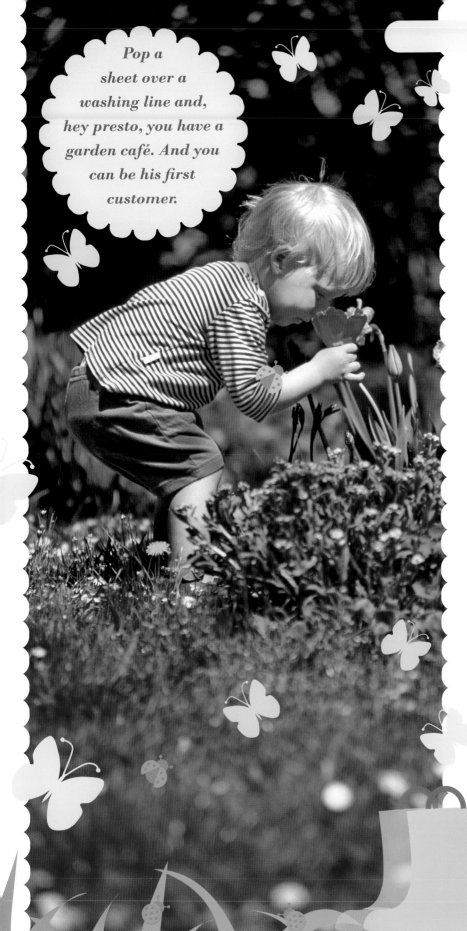

Pop a sheet over a washing line and, hey presto, you have a garden café. And you can be his first customer.

Get artistic

Art projects get a new lease of life when you get outside, since you have more space and mind mess a little less. Use chalk to draw roads and mazes on a pathway or patio, or race around each other's bodies in funny positions on large pieces of paper (lining paper is perfect).

Eat your greens

Grow quick-growing salad leaves that your child can pick and eat, or plant baby beets to be discovered and dug up like buried treasure. Local markets are wonderfully vibrant and noisy places to learn about fruit and vegetables; you can sample some snacks while you're there.

Grow your own giants

Plant sunflower seeds in small pots in spring and help your child water them. As they grow stronger, transfer outside and measure them together as they become taller than your child!

Bubbly personalities

Take bubbles outside where the wind will take them in unexpected directions. Some little ones prefer to chase them and pop them; others like seeing how long they can keep the bubbles up in the air.

The **10** golden rules

Your parenting skills really have a chance to shine in the toddler years. Here are some tried-and-tested strategies that (hopefully) will help you parent your toddler happily and effectively.

1
Remember she's a child

This might sound obvious but sometimes we forget our little ones are children not adults. Children have immature emotions and their cognitive skills, which help them think things through, are still developing. Remind yourself she is naturally egocentric, like all toddlers, and is not out to annoy you.

2
Praise, praise, praise

Your child loves pleasing you so acknowledging her achievements, such as picking up the toys, will make her want to repeat that behavior for yet more positive attention. Make sure you praise her for effort as well as achievement and you'll boost her self-esteem enormously.

Kids love routine. There'll be less need for conflict if they know what to expect at a particular time.

3
Ignore challenging behavior

As long as your toddler isn't hurting herself or another child, try ignoring any less appealing behavior. Giving attention to challenging behavior is a reward, of a kind. Tantrums are inevitable at this age, since toddlers can't express their frustration verbally so they act out.

4
Be consistent

Don't back down—she must know you mean what you say. Think three Cs—calm, clear, and consistent. Tell her exactly what you expect of her and warn her of the consequences if she doesn't do it and she'll eventually learn responsibility for her actions. Make your requests age-specific though, so she has a realistic chance of being able to achieve them.

5
Be a good role model

You are your toddler's most important teacher and she copies your model of behavior. When your patience is overly stretched, take a deep breath and speak gently but firmly to her instead of yelling. Show her how to be polite by demonstrating good manners yourself and try to stay calm in stressful situations.

DID YOU KNOW?

According to a University of California, Los Angeles survey, the average one-year-old hears the word "no" up to 400 times a day.

6
Make her feel important

Making your child feel important will encourage positive patterns of behavior. It's easy at times to let her chatter become background noise, but if you really listen to her, she'll feel heard and acknowledged. Focusing on her will help her cope with her emotions and make her less likely to throw a tantrum.

7
Choose your battles

Does it really matter if your child wants to wear odd socks or play for another five minutes in the bath? Your child needs to develop her own sense of self, and demonstrate her own taste and preferences. Let her know that anything to do with safety is non-negotiable, but if she "wins" on a few more trivial matters, it'll boost her sense of self-worth.

8
Distract to diffuse

Little children's moods can change quickly, which makes them easy to distract. Look out for signs that your child is getting to the end of her rope and distract her with her a toy or point out something if you're outdoors—"did you see the frog in the backyard?" Using humor can help, because it diffuses stress for you both.

9
(Don't) just say no!

Make an effort to not always stress the negative side of things. So, instead of telling your child what not to do, explain or show what she should be doing in order to nurture positive behavior. For instance, say, "carry the plate flat" rather than "don't tip the plate over." It will make life nicer for both of you.

10
Be realistic

Manage your expectations about your child's behavior. She's not being "naughty" when, for instance, she arches her back when you're trying to strap her in her stroller, nor are you an ineffectual parent. She's trying to assert her growing independence and asking for some control over her world; maybe she is ready to walk alongside you for a while.

Find the *fun* and the job's a *game*

One brush, two brushes, three brushes…

Brushing teeth, getting dressed, tidying up…in every household there is work to be done before playtime can start. With a little creativity, though, you can harness your child's enthusiasm while you cross off the chores.

(Don't) do it yourself

Resist doing everything for him. Your toddler loves mastering new skills and wants to do things himself. It may be quicker if you dress him, brush his teeth, and hold his hands under a running faucet, but he's probably ready to try. Patiently demonstrate what he needs to do then tell him how smart he is when he gets it right. Showing him he can do it himself increases his self-confidence and avoids daily flare ups.

Harness his helpfulness

Your child is at an age when he wants to help and please you, so nurture this urge by giving him little jobs to do. While you prepare food, ask him to arrange placemats on the table (however haphazardly) and witness his pride as he feels involved. Hang a row of hooks at his height for him to hang up his coat; praise him every time he does it.

Set a challenge

When he refuses to cooperate, set a challenge to intrigue his competitive instincts. Who is the champion tooth brusher, or will be first to find their shoes? Keep your challenges simple and let him win most of the time.

I've finished, I'm the fastest sweeper of all!

Get him in the habit

A two or three year old is not too young to have his own mini routine, and family experts believe it's important to get children involved in household tasks from a young age. Making a habit of putting his toys away, or pajamas under his pillow, builds self-confidence and instills behavior patterns now that will give him a sense of responsibility in years to come.

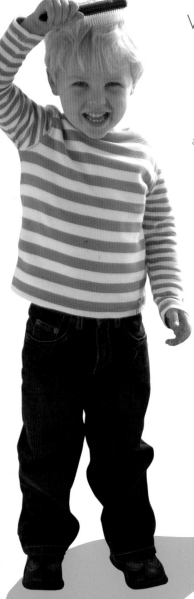
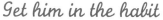

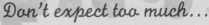

Natural copycat

Your toddler is a natural mimic—it's how he learns—and you are his number one role model. When you are putting on your shoes, encourage him to put his on at the same time. Eat breakfast together so he can see how you do it, and how long it takes you. Tidy up together at the end of the day. If you want to do some cleaning, give him a cloth and give him an area to dust. Don't expect great results but just appreciate the time this buys you to get a job done. He's learning good habits for the future, too.

Don't expect too much…

There will be some things that your toddler just can't do yet, so keep your requests simple and age appropriate. He might be able to put toys in a box, but putting books neatly on a shelf might be difficult. Be specific so he understands you: saying, "this room is a mess, tidy it up" might feel overwhelming to a toddler, whereas asking him to "put the bears on your bed" is more likely to get results.

I can clean like you, Mommy.

Magical make-believe

Your toddler's fantasy world is opening up, and there's endless scope for making mundane tasks more interesting. If he is bored in the supermarket, describe the shopping cart as a runaway train. Ask him to put on his boots so you can both go stomping in the puddles outside like explorers.

choo choooo

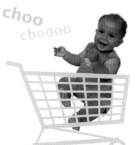

Put on some music

Distract him with music or nursery rhymes to get him through routine tasks that he regularly objects to, such as getting dressed or brushing his teeth. Creating positive associations will help him anticipate these fun moments and forget previous objections.

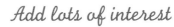

Add lots of interest

Your toddler's mind is buzzing and on the lookout for new experiences and information, so give him tasks that engage his brain. If you ask him to get some socks out of his drawer, ask him to find a different color every day. When combing his hair, ask him to count how many strokes you take, or if he would like to comb yours afterward.

What your child says
without speaking

Tying yourself in knots trying to grasp what your child is saying? You may well find actions speak louder than words.

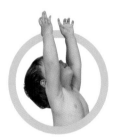

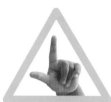

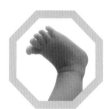

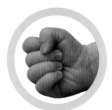

Do you speak "toddler" or "kiddish"? It's quite a skill, especially when the person you speak to has a restricted vocabulary, displays a warped sense of ego, is usually impatient, and can have anger management issues. Welcome to the world of translating a young child.

Quite often the way to communicate with your child is not through words at all, but through **nonverbal body language**. If you can decipher this, you will be able to understand more of what your child is telling you, and at the same time, help her to understand you better.

Babies use body language to communicate their needs right from the start: your baby might reach out her hand, point, touch, make eye contact, shake or nod her head, push something or someone away, or pull them closer. Psychologist and author David Chamberlain observes: "Both premature and full-term babies read faces so well that they can immediately imitate a wide-open mouth, a protruding tongue, or mimic expressions of happiness, sadness, or surprise." **Children are natural communicators.**

By two or three months, your baby can communicate with **a dazzling smile**. By 10 to 12 months, she might put your hand on the toy she wants to set in motion, she will lift her arms to ask to be picked up, and may **wave "bye-bye"** when you both say goodbye to friends and family.

As children get a little older, nonverbal language becomes more refined. They start to use single words or short sentences to emphasize meaning, while also using body language. Your child may point to a toy, and say "me play that," for example. As her attempts to use words increase, this can cause frustration when she isn't understood. You may see more body language as she expresses irritation, with pouting, hitting, crying, and stamping. The best way to avert these displays of frustration is to become skilled at **"reading"**

Tuning in to your child's growing repertoire of gestures and signs and showing her you understand is hugely rewarding for him as she sees her message getting through.

your child's unspoken language as it evolves. For instance, if a small baby averts her gaze, she's telling you she's overwhelmed and needs a break. An older baby, who has developed the capacity for self-conscious emotions, such as shame, might look away if she knows she's done something wrong. "When a young child refuses to look at you, it means she realizes that her actions may have disappointed you," observes psychologist Kristin Lagattuta.

If your child **covers her face** when she meets a new person, she's anxious, rather than rude. Similar actions might include chewing on clothing or hair, clutching your leg, or sucking her thumb. If your child is bouncing around, then she is ready to go outside, but if her shoulders are slumped and her movements are slow, it is time to rest and recharge.

You might notice your child using body language when with her peers. Babies and toddlers don't actually play with each other, but engage in "parallel play" where they play next to each other, often **mirroring each other's actions**. The body language involved complements language development and helps your child develop social relationships.

Given that your child is telling you so much without even speaking, what can you do to give her as much information as possible back again? Looking at your child is just as important as listening. Reply with visual cues, too. A **broad smile** when you are pleased will reinforce the message, as will **a shake of your head** when you say "No." Your child's auditory processing is much slower than yours and she needs **short, concise instructions combined with visual prompts**. "More juice?" as you hold up her cup works better than "Would you like some more apple juice in your sippy cup sweetie?" or "Aren't you thirsty?"

Using simple gestures or pictures will help your child **process information**. You could point to a picture of a bed in a book when you say "bedtime," or hold up your hand, palm outward, when saying "stop!" Some parents take this a step further by learning **baby sign language**, learning simple gestures for objects, emotions, and actions that both parents and child use. Some parents feel this really enhances communication whereas others worry it might delay speech.

Your stance, facial expressions, and tone of voice are how your child finds out what you are feeling and what you want from her, and being aware of this helps communication:

• **Use a smooth, calm voice** for normal, everyday talking. If you're scolding your child, use a firm but calm voice that lets her know you mean business. A harsh, angry voice will make her defensive, and can be difficult to decipher.

• **Make eye contact**. It shows she has your full attention, and increases the effectiveness of your message.

• **Sit or bend down to her level**, so you don't tower over her. Keep your arms open, rather than crossed, which can appear as hostile body language.

Keep communication simple: going at your child's pace will keep her switched on, engaged, and eager to communicate more.

Just as your child's facial expressions and body language can tell you what's going on inside her head, so yours tell her what she needs to know. A warm smile, a rub of her back, a wink… they all let her know you love her. And that's the most important message of all.

It's a question of
sleep

Your child's on the go all day, she must be tired and you need some shut-eye. So, why can sleep become an issue?

Why does my two-year-old still wake up so early?

This is one of the biggest complaints from parents. Your child needs about 11 hours or so of sleep each night, so if she's up with the rooster at 5 am, perhaps she's going to bed too early or napping too long during the day? Waking early may be her natural body clock but you can try to tweak it. A later bedtime might do the trick. Or if she still naps more than once in the day, try dropping a nap or, at least, ensure that she doesn't have a daytime nap any later than 4 pm.

How do I get her to "lie in" when it's so light in the mornings?

Make her room sleep-friendly with blackout blinds, and make sure she's not too hot or too cold. Try setting a night-light on a timer and tell her she should try to go back to sleep or be quiet until it comes on. And stuffed animal friends, and a handful of books near her bed can entertain her in the morning.

When should I move her to a bed?

Once she can climb out of the crib or you feel she's confident enough for a bed, then she's probably ready—usually between two and three years old. She's likely to be excited by the change, but if she's wary, praise her for being grown-up and make it a treat by letting her help you choose a new comforter cover.

What's a good bedtime routine now?

Young children like consistency so stick with your familiar routine. Bath, pajamas, teeth brushing, and a bedtime story in her room will make her feel warm and safe, and will be her cue for sleep. Keep to the same bedtime each night, too.

How do I get her to stay in bed all night?

For older, active children, nighttime wanderings can become all too familiar. If she comes into your room, just keep taking her back to her own bed, calmly and quietly until she breaks the habit.

Why does she find it harder to settle down when she's overly tired?

When your child is overly tired, it's harder for her to relax and to fall asleep, and she may also wake more at night. If you know she's worn out, start your bedtime countdown half an hour earlier.

Will siblings wake each other up if they share the same room?

Parents often worry about moving a young child in with an older sibling but it can help them both sleep well. Having someone else in the room and hearing each other's rhythmic breathing can be a comfort. Though, you'll need to plan two bedtime routines for quality story and cuddle time with both of them.

Sweet dreams, baby

As your child grows, her mind as well as her body becomes increasingly active, and her blossoming imagination—that's such fun most of the time—can bring on nightmares as she dreams up monsters and perhaps develops a fear of the dark. Quiet reassurance and soothing bedtimes can help counter fears.

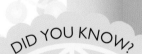

DID YOU KNOW?

Sleep is much more than simply a rest for the body, it plays a significant role in brain development and our brain's day-to-day ability to function. Scientific studies show getting the right amount of snooze time at night can be just as vital for a child's development as regular physical exercise and healthy eating.

 Too little sleep has been linked in studies to attention problems, bad moods, and even obesity.

Happy *talk*

The moment when your baby first says "mama" or "dada" is one to celebrate and cherish. But what will his next words be? And when will he be able to speak in sentences?

Every baby's language and speech skills develop at his own pace. In the first few months your baby will make cute cooing sounds and will be blowing salivary bubbles. By the age of three most children will have acquired a vocabulary of about 300 words and will be able to use simple sentences. Enjoy your child's attempts to grasp language—it is a fascinating insight into how speech develops.

Adults take for granted that we can make every sound that we need to express ourselves. But producing sound and speech is the result of a complicated and coordinated sequence of events involving the tongue, teeth, jaw, and palate, along with the vocal cords. Some sounds, such as "mmm" are easier to say than others, and will form the basis of first words. In addition to learning how to make noise, your baby's brain has to develop to be able to understand your language before he can start talking back. So, here's to the start of a lifetime of interesting conversations.

Whether he says "picy" (for "spicy") or "comsey" (for "clumsy"), record these endearing words since you'll soon forget.

Baby talk

Many parents-to-be swear that they will never use a baby voice, yet the reality is that everyone does—it's natural. "Motherese" (baby talk) is the singsong voice that parents use worldwide. Studies show that the high-pitch, simple vocabulary, short sentences, and exaggerated facial expressions help babies to engage and learn words faster.

I can hear you, Mommy!

The ability to communicate starts early: research shows that even when in the uterus a baby can recognize and respond to the sound of his mother's voice. From the minute they are born, babies assimilate information from the world around them and specifically from their parents.

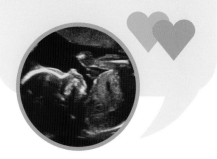

Doo-doo-doo-da-da-da

At three months your baby will start to babble and make vowel sounds, and by five months will add consonants ("goo-goo" or "ba-ba-ba"). Around 10–13 months, he'll point and say his first single words ("ball," "mama," "dada"), progressing to two-word sentences by 18 months ("Look plane!"). He'll love to talk to himself too, practicing his words.

I can speak clearly now

A two-year-old has a vocabulary of about 30–50 words, says three-word sentences (such as "Teddy is wet" or "Want more milk"), and he can follow two-step instructions from you. By the time he reaches three, your baby's vocabulary will include pronouns (I, me, you, and we). He'll start to talk more clearly, and you'll understand most of his speech.

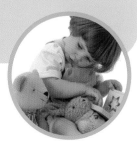

Nonstop talking

Hearing you talk is the best way for your baby to learn vocabulary and speech patterns and the more you do it the better. Keep up a running commentary of your day (from getting dressed and having breakfast to bath-time and bed) and talk to him as you do things together—it won't all make sense to your child but he will start associating these sounds with everyday objects and activities.

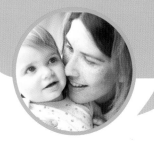

Look who's talking

Heading any self-respecting toddler's vocabulary is the word "No!" soon followed by "Why?" Nurture this inquisitiveness. When you are out ask him what he can see or point to things for him to identify. Instigate games such as spotting objects of a certain color or counting cars. You'll be surprised by what he can understand, recognize, and communicate back to you.

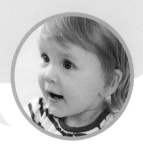

Toddlerisms

With increased language comes the inevitable "toddlerisms"—the endearing muddlings of words and tenses, the best of which can end up as part of your family lingo for years. He'll mix up words and make mistakes like "drawed" or "more bigger." Don't rush to correct him—confirm that you've understood him by repeating it back and smiling.

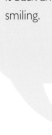

All in a day's play

Your child has an built-in curiosity and wants to explore the world with all five of her senses. There are many ways to indulge this, while also developing her creativity and giving her brain a bit of a workout.

Fun outdoors

Creepy-crawlies Head out into the backyard or to a local park on a bug hunt. Catching one and putting it (briefly) in a jar will give your little one the chance to learn more and examine the creature closely—how it moves, how many legs, where its eyes are. A magnifying glass may help.

Flower power Get your child to help you arrange some flowers that you have picked from the garden; then encourage her to notice differences in leaves, petals, colors, and fragrances.

Look at the sky Enjoy a warm day by looking for shapes in the clouds or discussing what patterns you see in leaves against the sky. Be as creative as you can and you'll fire your child's imagination and help it run riot.

Marvelous mess

Touchy feely Making art in a more tactile way adds an extra dimension of enjoyment. Try blobbing paint under plastic wrap to be smudged around, or adding food dye to corn syrup that you can mix and mess up—it dries wonderfully shiny, too.

Making tracks Foot- or handprints on T-shirts or laminated placemats make lovely gifts for grandparents, and are a good memento of your quickly growing child. Use water-based paints to ease the cleaning-up process.

Dough play Mix together two different colored doughs to make a rainbow dough—give her safe tools or things she can use to make an impression, or use cookie cutters to make different shapes.

Liquid or solid? Fuel your child's curiosity with this confusing mixture. Mix corn flour and water in a bowl to form a thick slime. Let it run through your fingers like water, then try smacking it, and feel the mixture turn solid beneath your hand. She'll be amazed as it switches from liquid to solid with a single movement.

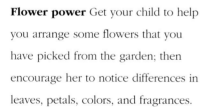

Making a mess is a great way to start your child experimenting.

How about that!

Sink or swim Gather a variety of objects and ask your child to guess which of them she thinks will float and which will sink; then test her predictions in a bucket of water.

Pump up the volume Bath-time provides great opportunities to make important discoveries about volume—just ask Archimedes. Give your little one a variety of containers of different shapes and sizes and encourage her to try pouring their contents from one into the other. Will all the water fit?

Treasure hunting Discover the power of magnets by using them to hunt for small metal objects in a tray of sand. You can also show her what the magnets do when you try to push them together.

Sun painting Put a small object, such as a key, on black paper and leave it in bright sunlight for a few hours. The rest of the paper will fade leaving a black outline, providing a graphic illustration of the sun's power.

Like oil and water Consider the significance of density by making a mini ocean. Fill a bottle half full with blue-colored water and top it off with cooking oil. Screw the lid on tight, then let your child play with it to discover that they don't mix.

Shapes & numbers

The shape of things to come Buy cookie cutters in simple geometric shapes and use them on a batch of pancakes or some dough. Talk about the shapes you make and compare them. Can you slot any together?

Simple subtraction Many of your child's favorite songs will hone her fledgling numerical skills and she will have fun learning them. Counting up songs, such as "This Old Man" helps with counting and basic addition.

Same same Something as simple as helping you pair the socks in the laundry can be a good foundation for mathematical concepts. Separating pairs of things (saucepan and lid, comb and brush) into two groups and asking your child to find its partner will help her see relationships.

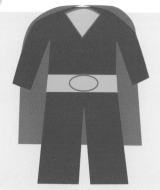
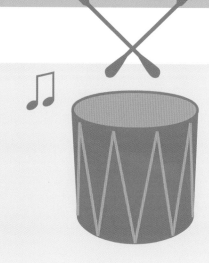

Stretching the imagination

Telling tales Test her creative writing skills before she can write: instead of reading to your little one, get her to tell you the story of one of her books just from looking at the pictures.

The puppet master Make simple puppets out of old socks with stick-on eyes, and put on plays with them. You could also snip the ends off gloves and decorate them to make finger puppets.

Costumes Encourage her to dress up in crazy clothes or costumes to take on other roles and personas—this both tests and advances her early acting and make-believe capabilities.

A picture paints a thousand words There are many exciting variations on simply painting a picture. Paint symmetrical butterfly pictures, print with bubble wrap, or draw a picture with glue and then sprinkle it with sand or glitter to add texture.

Art appreciation It's never too soon to take your little companion along with you to an art gallery; ask her to describe what she is looking at—you may find she has a totally fresh new perspective on what you are seeing.

Beautiful music Musical and percussion instruments can be made out of many household objects, or you may have a piano or a drum at home. Either way, encourage your little one to see what noises she can make.

Teddy Bear's vacation Stretch her imagination and play "let's pretend Teddy is going on vacation." Help her pack a bag of things Teddy will need and ask her to tell you where he is going, how he will get there, and where he will stay.

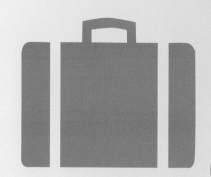

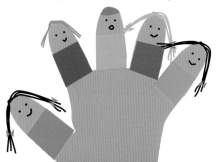

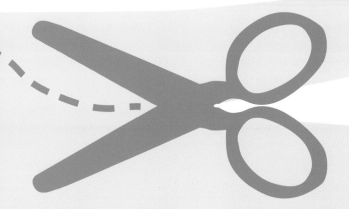

Always use safety scissors when cutting things with your child.

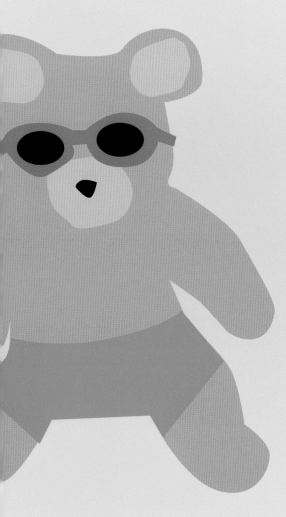

Using those hands

Cutting it Kids love to cut out shapes with safety scissors and stick them onto sheets of paper to make a collage. They also love to tear, so start her tearing up newspaper that you can use to stuff a paper bag that can then be used as an indoor ball.

In the bag Fill a freezer bag with clear hair gel, glitter, and foil confetti—your little explorer will love the feel of it as she squeezes, squashes, and moves the contents around to make a variety of different patterns.

Bejeweled Threading chunky beads together on a long piece of string is great for fine motor skills and encourages an eye for design.

Working it out!

Shake, rattle, and roll Fill plastic water or soda bottles with popcorn kernels, rice, or small pebbles, then slip them into a sock. Allow your little one to test out their different sounds before guessing what is inside.

Disappearing act Lay out a selection of items and then let her figure out which one you have taken away—this will sharpen your toddler's powers of observation, as well as her memory.

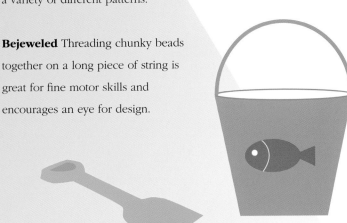

Driving you *potty?*

When your child is showing an interest in the toilet (other than to drop things in), grab the opportunity to start potty training.

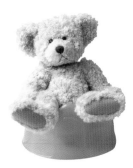

There comes a point when you have had enough of changing diapers: the cost, the washing, and trying to find a reasonable place to change your baby. Everyone seems to have an opinion about when is the best time to potty train, and what is the best method, yet every parent has to make up their own mind about when to start.

Attitudes toward toilet training vary around the world, and have changed even within recent generations. Before washing machines and disposable diapers became affordable and widely available, parents had every motivation to get babies out of diapers as quickly as possible. Young children were put onto the toilet or potties after every meal, and many were out of diapers by their first birthday. Advice about when best to potty train changed in the 1960s in the US and Europe when parents were advised to hold off until after 18 months.

Babies of the Digo people in East Africa are dry day and night by six months old.

In many countries early toilet training is still the norm, and one study estimated that 50 percent of the world's babies are **toilet trained by their first birthday**. Most parents in India, for example, consider it shameful to allow children to sit and sleep in their own waste. Western travelers on Indian transportation remark on the telepathic ease with which mothers hold tiny babies to the window to urinate. Chinese babies wear split-legged pants for easy squatting and early toilet training. Your grandparents might be amazed that contemporary children are in diapers for so long, although they may be impressed by the absorbent capacity of modern diapers.

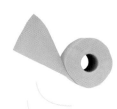

Advocates of **diaper-free parenting** (also called elimination timing) say babies can signal when they need to go from about four months old using gestures, sounds, facial expressions, and wiggling. Western parents used to be familiar with these signs, but with disposables there is no real sense of urgency, and this knowledge is not used. If you tune in to your baby and learn his cues, you can anticipate when to put him on a potty from an early age. You can encourage the link between **physical sensation and action** by talking to your baby from birth, and making urinating and grunting sounds so he knows how to tell you when he needs to go. The older the infant (over six months), the less likely he is to **recognize and signal the sensations**. Once your child becomes a toddler there are so many other distractions, timely communication can go a little haywire.

To try the elimination-timing method you must be **completely baby focused**. That means spending most days and nights at home with your baby while you develop intimate parent–baby communication. Once you know the signals you can teach these to your partner, family, and any other caregivers. If you need to do the school pickup, go to work, or care for another child, then this method may be challenging since it does take over your time in the early stages.

Most parents in the US and UK **toilet train** their children between **18 months and three years**. This is when most children develop the necessary bladder and bowel control. If your child becomes curious about you using the toilet, or starts to try to take off his own wet or dirty diaper, then this could be the right time for you to start training.

If you don't own any **potties**, buy one or two now so you always have one nearby; portable potties can be useful for when you're out. **Washable, cloth diapers** make a useful transition step since children who know how awful a wet diaper feels have a head start, so you could borrow some cloth diapers for a few weeks. Some toddlers love sitting on the potty whereas others find the adult expectation and gaze intimidating. The best approach is to **stay positive**, praise every successful attempt, and not fuss over the inevitable accidents. Though it's tempting to keep a toddler in diapers or training diapers while potty training, he'll get the message more readily if you keep him **diaper-free during the day**. Some children will urinate happily in a potty but might want a diaper back on for a stool; you might have to go with this for a while. Going half-naked around the home or backyard might help, as will using easy to pull up or down clothes. It's easiest to conquer potty training if you can stay at home for the first few days. When you have to head out, take changes of clothing, and expect to find yourself waiting while he sits in the park on his potty.

Babies "eliminate" about 20 times a day in their first weeks; this reduces to 10 times a day by three years old.

Toddler boys take an average one to three months longer than girls to get the potty habit, but this isn't always the case. Having an **older sibling** can mean that the whole process makes more sense, so this can make training quicker. Day-care centers also find they can train children quickly since the children notice others doing the same, and it becomes part of the usual routine. As your child gets the hang of it, provide a step so he can sit on the toilet. He might find it difficult to balance and reach toilet paper or wipes so don't be surprised if you have to help for a while yet. Start teaching a good **hand-washing routine,** too. Nighttime dryness comes later once your child develops further control over his bladder. Toilet training requires patience, humor, and self-confidence, and you will both get there eventually.

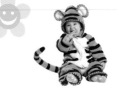

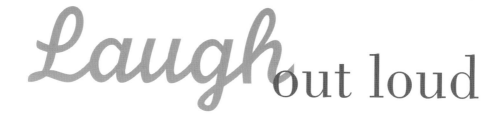

Laugh out loud

It's official—it's good to laugh. Everyone benefits from a good belly laugh and in more ways than one. By living with humor in her life, your child will learn how to bond with others and boost her self-confidence.

Discover exactly what tickles your child...

Let's get physical
Before your child's emotional understanding and verbal skills are sophisticated enough, her sense of humor is very much physical in nature—raspberries on her tummy will have her in fits, as will games, such as chase or peekaboo. "Row, row, row your boat," horsey rides on the knee, and being swung up into the air are sure to be hits.

Wait for it...
At about the age of two, her sense of humor is heightened by anticipation. So a song or game like "Pop goes the weasel" will have her in fits of giggles long before you get to "pop!" And her love of repetition means that however many times you play her favorite games or sing her favorite funny songs, she will always find them hilarious.

Get the job done
Humor is a great tool for managing your child's behavior and diffusing stress. If she won't put her toys away, for instance, appeal to her sense of humor—pretend to put the blocks away somewhere silly (say, up the front of your sweater), and with luck she will engage in the fun and show you where they really belong and need to go.

Oh-so slapstick
Visual humor is incredibly effective with toddlers and small children. Exaggerated parental "accidents" such as dropping things, or pratfalls will meet with hilarity—usually the sillier your actions, the stronger their reaction. Often just making silly faces or popping a funny hat on your head is all it takes to crack a smile or elicit a belly laugh.

Itsy bitsy elephant
By three, her speech and language skills are progressing rapidly and she'll love wordplay. Her sense of humor is now sophisticated enough to find it funny when you use the wrong words, so take old familiar songs and change the odd word for something silly, or make up rhymes with her name in it. Now who's up for "Itsy bitsy elephant" or a game of "hide and speak"?

You won't believe it!
Children don't inherit a sense of humor, it's learned from others. It doesn't matter if you aren't a natural comedian—just be willing to laugh at yourself and create a fun-filled, happy environment where your child feels safe to express herself. Children laugh about 200 times a day compared with just 15 times for adults, so encourage her to find the humor in day-to-day events and follow her cue for pranks.

On the same wavelength

In addition to trying to make your toddler laugh make sure you appreciate her sense of humor, too. Watch out for her "jokes" and respond enthusiastically—she will find them hilarious and will love it if you respond in kind. Understanding what makes her laugh will make you feel closer to her, and will boost her confidence as you allow her to take the lead. Most of all, nurturing her sense of humor reminds us that life should be fun.

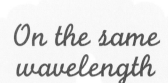

Laugh and the world laughs with you

Understanding humor is a crucial part of a child's emotional and social development. It teaches her how to socialize, handle disputes, and increases her self-esteem. Research shows that children with a well-developed sense of humor tend to be happier, more optimistic, and bond better with others.

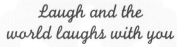

Natural differences

What makes boys so very different from girls? It's much more than DNA, it's due to the wiring in their brains.

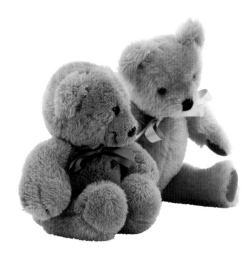

Talking with your friends at a playgroup, you watch one girl make a beeline for the dolls while a boy races around burning off energy. We've all heard the cliché about girls being different than boys, but is it true? Are they hardwired differently from birth, or do we make them different by how we treat them? It's the age-old **nature vs nurture** debate.

It's clear that boys' and girls' brains are **biologically different**. Hormones play a large part in this when, at around week six of pregnancy, the baby's sex is fixed. Boys receive a huge dose of male hormones—mostly testosterone—which affects their developing brain. Girls continue to develop without this hormonal boost, and although they will produce female hormones (estrogen and progesterone) these seem to have little influence on how the brain develops. Boys' brains tend to grow larger in general (about 12–20 percent), whereas some researchers have revealed that the region of the brain that controls language and emotion tends to be larger in girls.

From birth, baby girls are more **sensitive to touch** than baby boys and are more comforted by soothing words and singing. At just a few hours old, girls are more interested in people's faces than boys who are likely to be equally drawn to interesting objects. Baby girls tend to coo and gurgle at people. Most baby boys are equally chatty but are as likely to babble at a favorite toy as at a person. However, a study by the Institute of Psychiatry in London shows that only 3 percent of the variation in boys' and girls' speech development is due to their gender.

Even before understanding language, girls seem better at **recognizing emotions** in speech. One study of babies two to four days old showed that girls spent twice as long as boys keeping eye contact with a silent adult and also looked longer when the adult was talking. Boys' attention span, however, was the same whether the adult was talking or silent.

A baby boy has just as much testosterone as a 12-year-old boy. These levels drop a few months after birth, with a surge again at four years old.

As toddlers, girls usually display better **fine motor skills**, for example, holding crayons and pulling up zippers. Boy toddlers tend to like more **rough and tumble play** and they have 30 percent more muscle mass than girls, which might link to a need to run around. They can be more adventurous and are more likely to explore beyond the comfort zone of their parents. Boys can demonstrate a **better spatial ability** than girls, which means they're more attracted to 3D toys, such as footballs and building blocks, as well as moving objects, such as toy cars.

But how many of these apparent differences are actually related to biology and how many relate to how we as a society treat children? Some research argues that differences in boys' and girls' brains are soft- rather than hard-wired and that we're dressing up stereotypes—caused by how we treat children—as science. Are boys more attracted to building blocks because they are encouraged to play with them?

Gender stereotypes can be reinforced by parents, often unconsciously. For example, boys are more likely to be praised for being "brave" and girls for being "kind," so it can be easy for a parent to reinforce feminine or masculine stereotypes without making an active decision to do so. If you notice yourself doing this, try varying your approach. If your son loves climbing, great, but also nurture his quiet, focused side by sitting down and drawing with him or creating clay shapes. If your girl toddler loves books, remember to play ball games with her and praise her prowess on the jungle gym, too.

When **dressing a baby** it is hard to avoid the commercialization of gender stereotypes—little pink and blue outfits adorn the shelves of baby shops. Pink for girls and blue for boys seems ingrained in some cultures, yet for centuries both sexes wore the same clothes. When colored clothing came into fashion, pink was first associated with boys, and blue was favored for girls because it was the color associated with the Virgin Mary and femininity. This color coding switched over in the 1940s in Western Europe, so is actually a very recent fashion.

Gender stereotyping happens worldwide, but there are some historical and cultural exceptions. Girls in North American Indian tribes chop and carry wood just as much as the boys do and the women hunt buffalo alongside the men. **Cultural differences** can exist within a country too: African-American parents in the US, for instance, are less likely to stick to typical gender roles for their children whereas Mexican-American families are more likely to conform to traditional roles. In Sweden there is an active movement to discourage typical gender stereotypes, starting in kindergarten.

In Sweden, some kindergartens call children "friends" rather than "boys" and "girls" in an effort to break down gender stereotypes.

By treating your child as an individual, rather than defined by sex, you will help open up his or her world. Perhaps the reversion to type will happen anyway, but at least you can offer them the scope to choose. If you provide a stimulating environment full of opportunities, who knows what path they will take in life. It will be fun to watch.

Your child's inquisitive mind and

desire to explore the world will

give rise to a lifetime of

questions—the dreaded "why…?"

will become a recurrent theme.

I can do it,
all by myself.

Children appear to have an unquestioning confidence in their own abilities, which is why they get frustrated sometimes when they realize they can't do what they want to do. This also shows their determination to be independent, master new skills, and copy others.

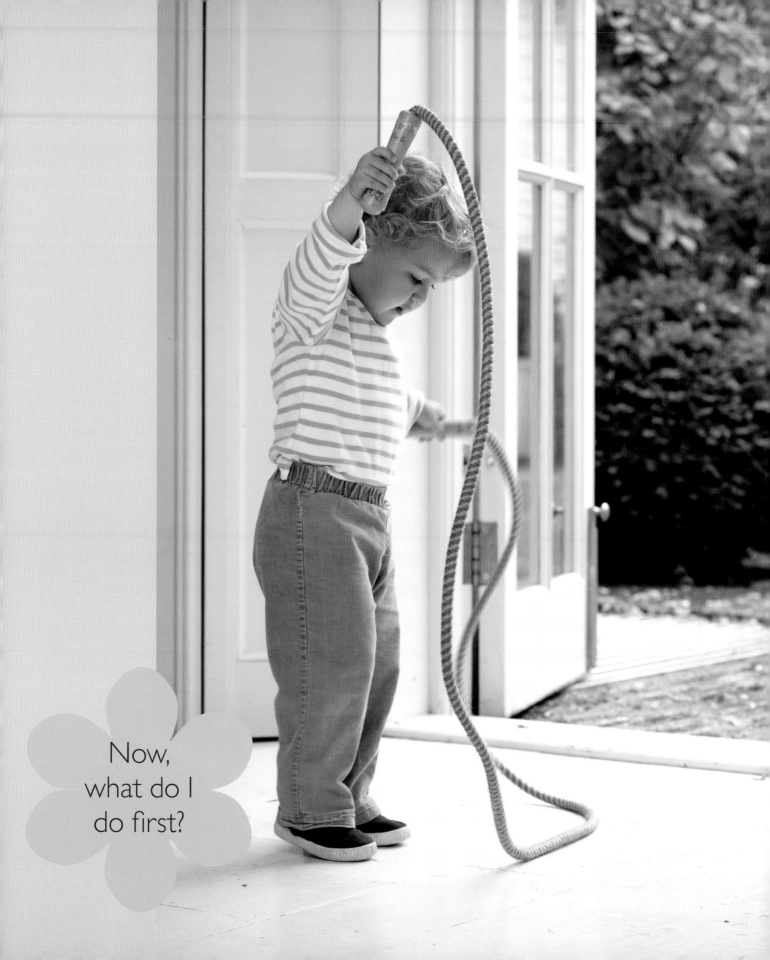

Now,
what do I
do first?

I am 3 years old

sleep

* 9–12 hours of sleep at night. May need one one- to three-hour nap.
* May start to be afraid of the dark.

food

* Has a growing appetite, and may have a favorite food.
* Needs at least five servings of fruit and vegetables daily, plus protein, carbohydrates, and fats.
* Uses a small knife and fork, but needs help with cutting.

teeth

* Has all 20 baby teeth.
* Learning to brush teeth, but will need help for a few years yet!

but why?

* Constantly curious, asking what, why, when, and where questions.
* Uses three- to four-word sentences, and can imitate five-word sentences.
* Has vocabulary of at least 300 words.
* Recognizes and communicates needs.

on the move

* Can balance on one foot for three seconds.
* Runs and turns quickly without falling.
* Rides and steers a tricycle and scooter.
* Jumps from low heights.

I can...

* Get dressed without help, and may be able go all day without a diaper.
* Hold a crayon and draw stick figures.
* Understand primary colors and name three shapes.
* Concentrate and listen actively to stories.

my world

* Expresses emotions, likes, and dislikes.
* Begins to show consideration for others and can be kind and gentle.

Look at me! I sing and talk, I run confidently, and I'm becoming increasingly more coordinated.

Your three-year-old loves lively family mealtimes. These social occasions provide positive interactions and conversation, and encourage good table manners as well as an enthusiasm for food.

Friendships flourish as your child matures socially and emotionally. He's starting to get a sense of other's points of view, shows empathy, copies caring behavior, and can take turns.

How can I help? Toddlers love to feel important and involved. Give him small tasks, such as helping sort laundry, mailing a letter, or washing his plastic cups.

It's a boy! Children start to identify gender now, labeling themselves and others (not always accurately). They may "gender type" clothing and toys, whether or not you've encouraged it!

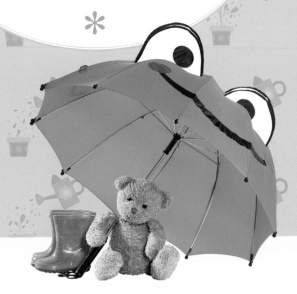

You're *one* of the *family*

As your child starts to be aware of other people as distinct from herself, she will also begin to have a sense of her family and where she fits into it.

Families these days come in all shapes and sizes, and your child may start to notice that not every family is exactly the same. **Nuclear families** with a married mom and dad living together with their own biological children are still the most common around the world, but this is changing. In the US, nuclear families make up about 4 in 10 families, a figure down more than 20 percent since 1960. A survey in 2012 showed that there are **35 different kinds of family structure** including step, single parent, and blended (children from different relationships brought up together).

Family size is changing too, with a predominance of smaller families than in previous generations, when up to ten children was not uncommon. Today, many families are small units with one parent and one or two children, whereas in others the extended family plays a growing role. With parents working long hours or even overseas, **extended family,** such as grandparents, take on the key caring role. **Matriarchal societies** feature women doing the child rearing together, with men earning money, and in some African cultures a child may be unaware of her biological parents but thinks of a range of adults as being "hers."

Your own view of **what "family" means** may change now that you are a parent. You may look at your own childhood and family life in a different light, and question how you want to **raise your own children**. Perhaps a traditional model is important to you, or maybe you prefer more alternative methods. Hidden hopes and concerns may come into play: if one of your parents was absent, you may want the opposite for your child, and make it a priority in your **life choices**. Whatever you choose, your child will grow up accepting your family model as the norm, and it will be completely natural to her.

21st century family life

✳ Make your family bond strong from the beginning by making at least one day a week a "family day." Eat together, do activities as a family, and have plenty of time to putter around doing nothing together.

✳ 14 percent of families in the US and 24 percent in the UK consist of a single parent. There are lots of support networks for single parents where you can meet for practical and emotional support, socializing, and arrange shared vacations with other single-parent families.

✳ An estimated 240,000 children in the US live with same-sex parents. In the UK, one in 111 families has gay, bisexual, or transgender parents.

✳ Families often now live farther away from loved ones. A large number of US families today are based more than 100 miles from their own parents. Use Skype and social networks to keep in touch between visits.

{ *If your child has cousins, make an effort to get them together as often as is possible. By growing up together from an early age they will all have the earliest and closest memories of each other, and these can develop into strong adult family relationships.* }

✳ If extended family is going to play a key role in raising your children you all need to agree to diplomatic ground rules about how to make important decisions, who does which jobs, and how to communicate with day-care and school. Make sure there is time for them to have fun together too, rather than just day-care pickups and child-care tasks.

Character *building*

What kind of person will your child turn out to be? Like you?
Like your partner? Or a totally unique and new character?

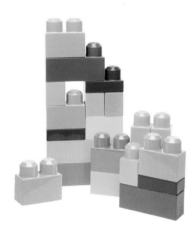

The famous quote "Give me a child until he is seven and I will give you the man" implies that early childhood defines the person your toddler will become. Many parents say that their child's personality was evident from day one: he wiggled in the uterus and is now just as active as a toddler, or that he had a sassy smile as a baby and continues to have a sassy sense of humor. Is your child born with his personality set in stone, or does it have more to do with the way you raise him? If you think your child might inherit your grumpiness, or stubborn nature, can you, or indeed should you, do anything to influence how he "turns out"?

> The age-old debate about nature vs nuture continues. Is your baby born with his personality or can you influence how he turns out?

There has been a lot of research about whether a child's character is predetermined by an **inherited set of genes,** or if environment and experience have more influence. The World Health Organization cites research that says the care and stimulation a child receives in the first two years affects his brain development. There is a growing consensus that no single factor is solely responsible for how we develop, but rather that both **genes and upbringing shape personality**.

It's easier said than done, but resist the urge to label your child as "shy," "bubbly," or any other **personality cliché** since very few children are always one way or the other. The calmest child can have a lively day, and a gregarious child will also enjoy some quiet time. What might be considered an outgoing child in one family, may be considered reserved in another. Feeling that your child is judged or labeled as a particular personality trait can ruffle the feathers of any parent. If someone comments that your child is shy or a chatterbox, for example, rephrase this in a more positive way, with: "he is a real observer," or "yes, he is very friendly."

Many parents express a desire for their children to be more confident than they were themselves as a child, or more studious, but **can you influence** how your child is? Some experts believe that certain temperaments make it easier to encourage your child along a particular path. If your toddler is laid back and receptive to new situations, you may have an easy time nudging him in a certain direction, for example, to join a singing group or to try a new sport. However, if your child is reserved in new situations, pushing him in a new direction may increase his wariness more.

Is there an age when **character traits** become fixed? It's possible that the early years provide an important window of opportunity for your child. One 2010 study reported in *Life Science* suggests that a child's character is set by the age of six. It followed 2,400 children from the 1960s and compared teacher "personality" reports with character traits 40 years later and found that these same traits influenced their behavior as adults. Other studies show more variety, and suggest that **personalities do evolve over time**, shaped by life events and external influences.

Research published in 2010 reinforces the theory of the interaction between genes and environment, noting how effective parents take a **child's nature** into account when making day-to-day decisions. You can help an overly boisterous child recognize boundaries, and a socially awkward child find ways to play with others. Nathan Fox, a human development professor at the University of Maryland, believes that while your child's temperament can dictate how social situations play out, paying attention to "temperament" cues avoids distress and can **build your child's confidence**. Being sensitive to your child's particular traits can help you predict what will or won't work for him and can help a reserved child to flourish. Fox warns against being overly protective and suggests that gradually exposing a child to new social scenarios with you at his side can help him overcome fears and become more socially confident. You can also help your child to develop conversational strategies, for example try teaching him to say, "Can I play that game with you?"

Your child could have a gene for being artistic, but you need to provide the paper and paint and take him to art museums.

The latest research says that certain genes may be turned "on" or "off" by a particular **environment**. A stressful, chaotic home may activate a gene for shyness, while that same gene remains dormant in a calm home. It follows that while your baby's genes may favor him having certain traits, for example, being friendly or creative, he needs to be in a stimulating environment for these traits to flourish.

Social and emotional support are important, but practical care and nutrition have a bearing too. Tired, hungry children will be irritable, no matter what their natural temperament is and a nutritious, varied diet will help keep your child calm. A safe, comfortable home will help your child feel secure and foster his confidence that the world is a good place to explore.

There's little doubt that your child's **early years** are formative for his emerging personality, and your role is key. And it will be lots of fun to see how he turns out.

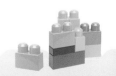

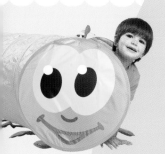

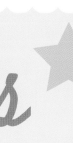

Making *friends*

As your child grows, she'll start to make friends. From compromising and sharing to having fun, there is plenty to learn from others her age.

Children like playing with other children because it's fun, pure and simple. So, what's the best way to encourage your child to make friends? The most important thing is give her the chance to meet and socialize with other children—take her to the park, meet up with friends and their children, go to playgroups, perhaps enroll her in a preschool a couple of mornings a week, and nurture her relationships with other children in the family. Then, as much as possible, let her play! It's tempting to try to steer things, but friendships need space to develop naturally rather than be forced.

Playing with others

Play is an essential part of childhood and it's how children learn myriad skills, including cooperation, taking turns, and new ways to do things. From about 18 months, toddlers engage in associative play—playing loosely with others, perhaps as a game of chase—but it's not until about three years old that children enjoy cooperative play and work as part of a team, for example, to build a tower of blocks.

To encourage her associative and cooperative play, if you have a child over for a playdate try to think about how to get activities started. You could put out games such as floor puzzles or blocks, or a big sheet of paper with crayons or paints for each child and sit them next to each other.

Your child's personality

Tailor activities to suit your child's personality and energy levels each day—if she's tired or feeling reserved a noisy soft play center or playgroup may be overwhelming. Playing at home with one friend may be much more enjoyable for all.

It's understandable to be frustrated if she's being shy and not joining in, but it doesn't matter at this early stage. Some children form attachments with one or two friends, whereas others thrive on playing with lots of different children. Acknowledge any anxieties and gently encourage her to socialize in her own time. Try not to say "don't be silly," since this sounds dismissive

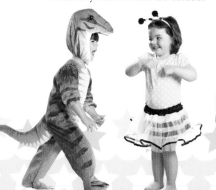

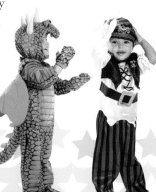

of her concerns. Equally, resist apologizing to other adults for a trait such as shyness; just say she'll be fine in half an hour when she's used to the new surroundings and people.

Sharing and turn taking

Sharing is a tricky concept for your child—she lives in the moment and wants everything now. Being told she can have a toy in 10 minutes means

Be a friendly role model

Children learn how to behave and interact with others from adults, so let your child see you being relaxed and friendly with people and treating them with respect. Smile and say "hello", and your child will learn that this is the best way to act.

If you were a timid child or are a reserved adult, try not to project your feelings or reservations on to her—

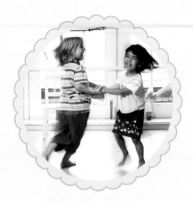

Play boosters

Play games with your child that involve taking turns and sharing. She will learn that it's fun to play even if she doesn't always get her own way.

★

Encourage her to take risks that will boost her self-confidence and her play skills—for example, let her master a toddler jungle gym without you hovering nearby.

★

Praise your child when she plays well with others, and be specific, for example, "you took turns with your scooter very well."

★

Keep playtime with other children short or have a break for a drink and a snack to keep energy levels up. Bad behavior may be triggered by hunger and fatigue.

> Elephants, dolphins, chimpanzees, and bats have been shown to form life-long friendships like humans.

nothing to her—she can't tell time yet and it requires advanced social skills to empathize with others. Just assure her that it will be her turn afterward, or you could use a timer so she knows when it's her turn.

Try only to intervene if she (or another child) is getting upset and she can't resolve the conflict herself, or if you need to address her behavior. Snatching toys or hitting will stop other children from playing with her, so she will need prompt help to stop this behavior. If she's squabbling, take the toy from her and say calmly, "It's Tom's turn now."

she may be completely different than you. If you lead by example and show that it's good to talk happily to others, she will do her best to copy you.

Do you like her friends?

It can be tricky if you and your child are drawn to different people. Keep an open mind unless a child is hurtful toward her, in which case steer her to play with others. You may not always like the behavior of your friends' children, and your child won't always play nicely with children you do like. Don't make an issue of it—being nonjudgemental is another positive message for your child to learn.

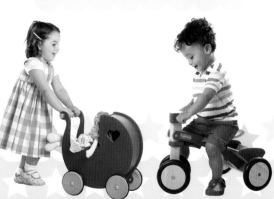

Make friends, make friends, never, never break friends…

Children are protective of their things, so don't expect her to share a favorite toy.

Actively playing with other children means having to learn to share. And this takes time! Lead by example and use positive encouragement. This key skill helps her to socialize easily, enabling real friendship to grow.

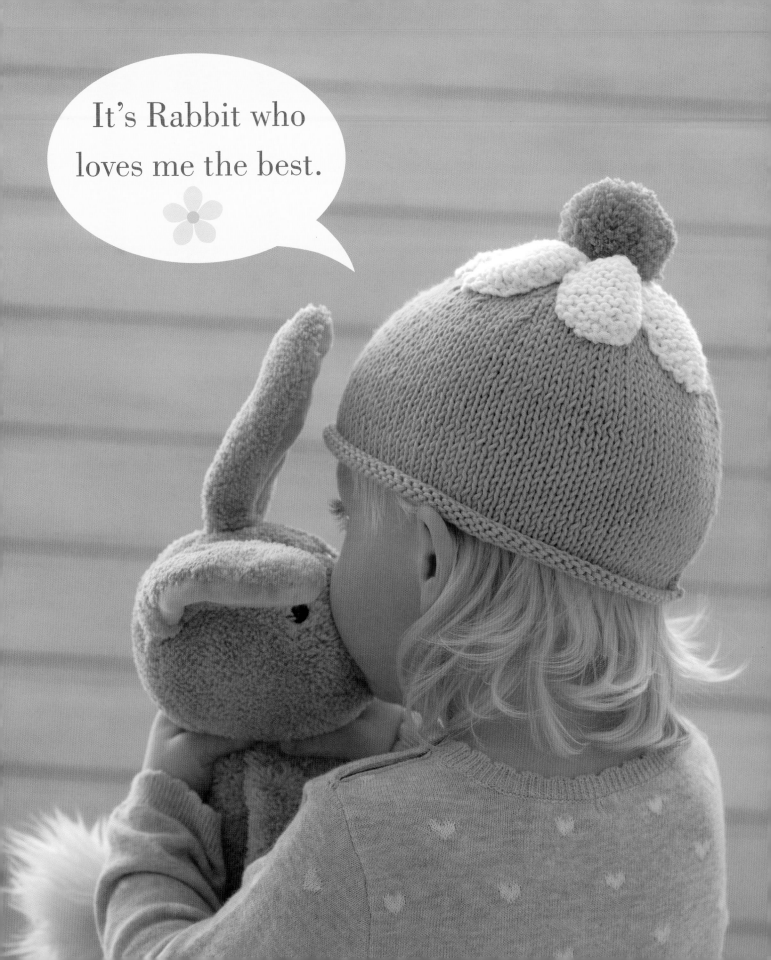

Your *little helper*

Your baby is growing up and starting to want to do things for himself. Are you ready for this burst of enthusiasm?

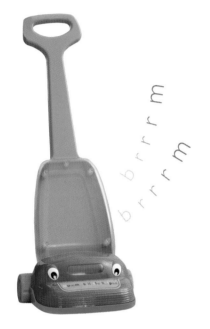

brrrm brrrm

Y**ou have spent the last year or two** fetching and carrying for your child: picking up socks, brushing teeth, making meals, putting away plates…. But at some point your child will need to do more himself, both for your sake and for his. How do you manage the transition from doing everything for your child, to encouraging his independence? Unless you want to be washing him into adulthood, you need to introduce him to what he can do for himself, and make it enjoyable.

From the age of **18 months**, your toddler will experiment with becoming more independent, toddling off now and then to explore on his own, most happily while you're sitting firmly rooted to one spot so he knows where you are if he feels scared. **Curiosity and the desire for independence** tip the balance over his need always to be close to you.

You are more likely now to hear: "No! Me do it!" as your child wants to attempt to do more things for himself. Coming up to **three years old**, improved **coordination and body control** mean he is much more capable of doing complex tasks, such as feeding himself, getting undressed, and putting away toys. Even so, his desire to "help" you and do tasks for himself will most likely outweigh his skills. Your toddler might want to carry his cup of water, but it might not make it to the table without spills every time. He wants to please you, but at the same time wants to assert his ideas and opinions, so while baking seems like a fun activity, washing his hands before and afterward might not be so popular.

It is tempting not to indulge these attempts to join in, especially if you value a tidy home or time is limited, but **toddlers love helping**, and the discouragement that comes from being passed off or restricted can lead to tantrums, family discord, and a crushed spirit. Offer **praise and encouragement**, and reign in the urge to do the task more quickly and

Chores celebrate a child's accomplishments and help him feel like a full participant in family life.

expertly. You might need to reschedule parts of your day to allow more time. Encourage your **child's initiative** now and it's more likely to stick into the preteen years, when children can be incredibly helpful around the home.

Your toddler wants to help with the laundry and cooking? Great. It's what he's designed to do as a growing toddler, and what he needs to do to develop his motor, emotional, and social skills. He's picking up cues from you and his environment and trying to put them into action, and learning how to become part of the world he's now more aware of. Being able to **accomplish an "adult" task** boosts a child's confidence in mastering the world around him and shows him that independence is achievable rather than scary. It raises his expectations of what he can expect of himself and how he can contribute to **family life**. Getting things wrong is inevitable but it builds resilience and the ability to make good judgements, both of which are essential to your child's **psychological well-being** when he starts making forays into playgroups and at school. Letting go of a little parental control and allowing your child to explore how things work in a safe way is good for you, too, offering much-needed practice for the years to come.

When should you expect children to be capable of helping usefully? That depends on where the child is raised and by whom. Toddlers of the Kipsigi people in south-western Kenya are routinely given real household chores from two years old, so that by six they are playing a full role in providing and caring for the family. In villages across India, four-year olds are learning the rudiments of agriculture

and girls have domestic chores, having been introduced to the tasks as toddlers with weeding and taking care of siblings.

So what kinds of tasks are **good starter activities** for this age group? Research suggests these should be achievable: getting undressed and into pajamas, brushing teeth, and tidying toys or putting away crayons. Toddlers especially like chores involving "grown-up" items: piling laundry into a basket, getting a clean diaper when you're changing the baby, collecting fallen leaves with a mini rake, and finding the family shoes and lining them up. Are there jobs that he can be in charge of? Expect to **supervise every activity** at first, and to keep up the reminders, tips, and praise. Your child will get distracted, and there may be more mess after the chore than before, but there are practical ways to encourage him to help and make the process less work for you—put up a row of hooks at child height for his coat, keep a drawer in the kitchen for his cutlery, and position boxes at an accessible height for tidying up DVDs, blocks, and toys. Research suggests offering to pay pocket money or other rewards doesn't pay off in the long term.

The best predictor of young adults' success in their mid-20s was that they participated in household tasks when they were three or four.

Studies suggest that a household routine that includes regular chores **strengthens family relationships**, makes children feel secure, and leads to increased well-being, which lasts into young adulthood. Chores weave your child into the routines of the household, providing a predictable structure that seems to support early development and a happy family life.

It's a wonderful life

With a plethora of parenting advice available at the touch of a button and spilling off the shelves, it's worth zoning out at times and embracing your own amazing journey into parenthood and family life.

Your unique family

Above the general "parenting" chatter, the message from many child experts is that there is no ideal family, no one right way to raise a child. It's music to the ears to hear that the key to making it good as a parent is actually fairly simple, and that it's OK if we all do it in a slightly different way, finding what's right for us, shaped by our own experiences, cultural heritage, and upbringing.

Studies show that what's important is that we are "good enough" parents, providing nurturing food, comfortable shelter, and love—and beyond these, consistently responding to a child's needs. How you achieve this is up to you and your own personal preferences—whether you breast- or bottle-feed, use a front carrier or a stroller. Being responsive is so much more than these everyday practical choices—it's about reading and responding with love and care to your child's cues in the way that feels most natural, questioning your responses, and treating your child as an individual.

On-the-job training

With no preset rules and with each family having its idiosyncracies, possibly your most valuable parenting asset is your gut instinct. When this wavers, it's fine to stumble a little as you figure out the next best step to take, gain another insight, and recognize increasingly that this is an unpredictable journey on which you need to adapt to changes and evolve. You haven't missed a trick—picking your way through this parenting journey is simply part of the fun.

All together...

While centering on your child feels so right, it's worth taking a holistic approach to family life. Children are especially effective barometers of mood, and a happy, relaxed couple is more likely to transmit these sentiments to their child and provide effective and nurturing parenting.

Husband-and-wife psychologists, Carolyn and Philip Cowan, stress how prioritizing your own well-being and your relationship with your partner is key to how children fare both emotionally and socially.

The rewards

While nurturing your child is an immeasurable task, contemplating the rewards is deeply reassuring. The unconditional love and admiration you receive can blow you away, as you realize that to him you are the bravest, strongest, and best, and can wash away all his woes with a simple hug. Life takes on new dimensions as you get the chance to be a child again, rediscover simple pleasures, and create your own special family.

Your life has expanded, never to be the same again—scary, but oh-so exhilarating!

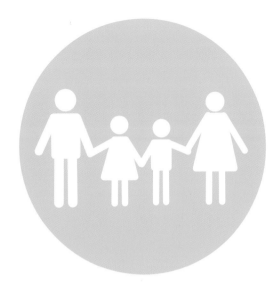

Expanding your *family*

Thinking of another baby

You've just got the hang of life with a young child and you might even be getting a good night's sleep, so it might be time to have another baby…

I f thoughts about a second baby have started to flit through your head, you're already gearing up psychologically for the **adjustment** this would involve. There are many factors to consider. Is your partner thinking along the same lines? In addition to being exciting, a new baby inevitably brings added stress, including sleepless nights and a demanding feeding regimen. Are you ready to embrace this together and be **mutually supportive**? And do you feel **financially ready** to expand your family? Then there is your first child to consider. Do you have a preferred age gap? You may want to deal with the tiring baby years close together, and think siblings **closer in age** will have more in common; or perhaps you feel in need of a break and think a bigger age gap gives siblings more **independence**. If you had trouble conceiving the first time you may want to start trying soon, especially if age is a factor—although this means running the risk of getting pregnant immediately, which may not have been in your game plan either.

It's just as important the second time around to feel **fit and healthy**. Optimize your chances of conceiving by eating a **nutritious, balanced diet**, avoiding alcohol and limiting caffeine consumption, and drinking plenty of water. Remember to start taking any necessary supplements, such as folic acid (see opposite). Are you energetic and relatively fit, or could you lose a bit of lingering pregnancy weight? Getting yourself in shape will help give you the stamina you need for the **journey ahead**.

Did you know?

✳ A healthy intake of omega-3 fatty acids found in oily fish, such as salmon, can boost the development of a baby's brain and nervous system, and may reduce the chance of a baby developing eczema.

{ *The critical time for taking folic acid supplements (400 mcg daily) is three months before conceiving and during the first three months of pregnancy. Folic acid helps the healthy development of a baby's brain and spinal cord.*

✳ Snacking on dried apricots gives your iron levels a helpful boost in pregnancy—one small handful provides 10 percent of your daily iron needs.

✳ Calcium found in dairy products and fortified orange juice is a top pregnancy nutrient, contributing to the healthy development of your baby's bones, teeth, muscles, heart, and nerves.

✳ A rainbow of fruit and vegetables carries an impressive nutritional punch, providing fiber, antioxidants, and a whole range of vitamins and minerals, perfect for optimizing fertility and providing essential nutrients for a growing baby.

✳ If, like many people, you use sunscreen, you might need a vitamin D supplement. A growing body of researchers are calling for pregnant women to take supplements of vitamin D just as they do folic acid, since it is essential for a baby's development.

Does *birth order* matter?

Is the eldest child always the most serious? The youngest the most gregarious? And is there really a "middle-child syndrome"?

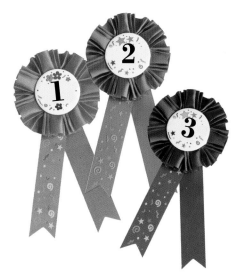

When you look at your toddler, it's hard to imagine the person she will become. Could she be the next president or an international CEO? A great writer or painter? A rock star or concert violinist? According to some psychologists, your child's personality and who she will grow up to be **may be influenced by the order** in which she is born into your family. Is it by chance that so many US presidents, British and Australian prime ministers, and other world leaders are firstborns, as are pioneering artists, such as Barbara Hepworth and Pablo Picasso? Or that revolutionary thinkers, such as Aung San Suu Kyi, René Descartes, and Nicholaus Copernicus, have been last-borns? Or that adept social animals, such as Madonna and David Letterman, are middle-born children?

The importance of birth order is a **hotly debated topic** by psychologists. According to theory, the **typical firstborn personality** is high-achieving, hard-working, reliable, responsible, and a good leader, if somewhat conventional and uptight. This may be why studies seem to show that firstborns are more likely to end up in leadership roles. An eldest child is closest to the parents in many ways, and can also act as surrogate parents to younger children, which reinforces this role.

By contrast a **typical youngest child** may be fun-loving, creative, adventurous, and rebellious. She may not have the eldest's authority but she knows how to turn on the charm. Her special place as "baby" of the family may make her more outgoing and social than your eldest but also leads to the risk of her becoming spoiled and dependent as an adult.

Firstborn and last-born children are in a special position since they will both benefit from some **one-on-one parenting time** that can have a positive effect on their IQ. But does this mean that middle children lose out? **Being in the middle** can be positive: they seem to make up for the difference in

> ## Parents spend an average 25 minutes more quality time each day with a firstborn child than a second child of the same age.

family attention by making an extra effort outside the family, and they are often good team players and negotiators. The term "middle-child syndrome" refers to middle children who feel neglected, have low self-esteem, and can be attention-seeking as they try to carve out their place in the family.

Children may seek to **carve out a different identity** depending on their siblings. If your firstborn is an academic high-flyer, for example, your next child may find something else in which to excel. And research shows that firstborns tend to be the brainiest sibling. A Norwegian study published in the journal *Science* showed that eldest sons tended to be 2.3 IQ points higher in score than those who were second born, and that this trend continues down the line. This may seem insignificant, but it could translate into the difference between getting into a top university or not. A 2011 study by an American careers website found that firstborns and only children were more likely to bag a senior level position in a company, such as CEO, and more likely to earn a six-figure salary than later-born children.

So, can you **help your kids thrive** whatever their birth order? You may want to treat all your children in exactly the same way, but this is not always possible or appropriate given they will have **different personalities and needs**, and you may simply have less time. You can help your eldest relax a little by reassuring her that everything does not have to be perfect all the time and that she can learn from her mistakes, and by not piling on the responsibility. And don't pamper your youngest; let her stand on her own two feet and nurture her toward independence. It's easy to underestimate what youngest-born children can do. Conversely, other families find that they overestimate their child's ability, comparing it with what big brother or sister could do at the same time. Try to resist this, and save any comparisons for when your youngest cannot hear. And for your middle child, give her that special one-on-one time and make an effort to take her to activities without her siblings so she develops her own interests.

> ## Later-borns may be risk takers. A study of brothers playing baseball showed that younger brothers were ten times more likely to steal a base and were also three times more likely to succeed.

The person your child will become depends on a complex interplay between the genes she inherits and the **culture and opportunities** she is exposed to both inside and outside the home. **Gender, age gap, and the family finances** can all make birth order less important. **Gender** may reduce the birth order factor in that children of different sexes may already feel different and feel less need to "compete." **Child spacing** also has an effect. If you have a second child after five or six years, you effectively have another firstborn. **Money** is a factor since it can mean that siblings may not get the same opportunities. Younger children may have more money spent on them, especially if they are the last one to leave the family nest.

There is no magic recipe for giving your eldest, your middle, your youngest, or your only child the perfect start in life—as a parent you can only do your best to balance your different children's needs, starting with giving them each plenty of your love, time, and attention.

Pregnant
with toddler in tow

The days of pampering yourself during pregnancy may seem a distant memory when you already have a rebellious or rambunctious older child. Yet with planning and help, this can be a special experience, too.

Save your energy

Be easy on yourself. If your toddler still naps, take a nap yourself. Quiet activities like reading, arts and crafts, and jigsaws puzzles may keep him happy while you lie down next to him. Try sofa-based games, such as "dog-indoors"—you lie on the sofa and throw something he can fetch; indoor treasure hunts or playing doctor also work well.

Burn his energy

Make sure you give him lots of opportunities to let off steam. Take him to the park, soft play areas, or the playground. Play active games such as "Simon says…" —you sit and relax while issuing energy-burning orders, such as making him do jumps, race long distances between trees, or find certain items for you, such as a stick or leaf.

Enjoy rainy days

Wearing out your toddler may be more challenging if the weather is miserable. But visiting the library, or even a museum or art gallery for older kids, or catching a kids' movie is a way you can both get out and have fun, too. Soft-play centers and swimming pools are also good—plus the buoyant water will help support an aching belly.

Help build up independence

If your older child isn't yet toilet trained, wiping his own bottom, dressing himself, or sleeping through—tackling these issues now (as appropriate to his age) may save you a lot of pain later. Motivational tactics such as stickers and reward charts can work wonders with older children.

Feeding the hungry hordes

Pregnancy and a toddler means it's constant feeding time. Batch-cooking healthy meals in advance and freezing some may help you stave off hunger (and fatigue), and you can employ your toddler's help to give him an activity, too.

Accept help

If family and friends offer help with chores or child care—take it! Striving to do everything perfectly yourself is stressful, so swallow your pride, accept help, and lower your standards on housework for while.

Buddy up

Arrange regular playdates with other friends, ideally outdoors. You and your friend can sit and catch up while the kids happily tire themselves out together.

Outsource as much as possible

If you can afford it, pay for it. Modern living means we don't always have community to fall back on, so pay for a cleaning person, a babysitter, or someone to do the ironing. If your toddler is already in child care, you might want to consider keeping him there some of the time—to give you a rest and to keep up his social and educational development.

Get ahead with the internet

The internet is a boon to tired moms, saving you time and precious energy. Order groceries online, but also save stress by getting ahead on things such as friends' birthday presents and school uniforms for older kids.

Visiting the doctor

A reluctant toddler may not be your ideal companion for routine doctor appointments, but taking your older child along demystifies it for him, too, so that hopefully the reality of a new baby will start to sink in, and he won't find the idea of you having a baby too scary. Take along a coloring book, crayons, and healthy snacks, with maybe even a promise of a tasty treat as a reward for good behavior—this may ease the process for you both.

Preparing them and you for birth

Babies can be boring—manage your toddler's expectations so he isn't disappointed when baby sister does nothing but eat, sleep, and cry. Cuddling up and reading picture books about having a new baby can help prepare them. Enlisting your toddler's help in preparations can keep him busy and spark enthusiasm, for example, asking him to help you sort old toys for the baby is hours of fun for him, too.

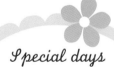

Special days

These days alone with your toddler will never be repeated, so make the most of this precious time. Take him out and have fun together, before your next little one arrives. Hopefully he will remember how special he is to you when some months down the line the realization sinks in that the new baby actually takes up a phenomenal amount of your time… and is here to stay.

Hello
I'm your big brother

A sibling is a wonderful gift to give your child, and a new baby is exciting for the whole family. It may take a little while to adjust to your new family setup, but sibling rivalry isn't a given and there are steps you can take to make the transition a smooth one.

All change

Children are creatures of routine and they don't like surprises, so preparing your older child for the new arrival is a key part of helping him adjust to the change. Perhaps wait until you have a real belly and can feel the baby moving before you tell him about the pregnancy, so that it is more real. He's got no concept of time so put the due date in context for him, such as just before his birthday or after Christmas. Share books together about the arrival of a new baby and introduce him to other babies in the family. Make him feel involved right from the start by letting him help you sort out his old clothes and instill future closeness by saying "our baby" and "your baby sister" instead of "the baby."
When baby arrives, try to continue your older one's daily routine as much as possible since consistency will make him feel secure and calm. If he's at preschool, take his sibling in for "show and tell"—he'll enjoy showing her off.

Musical beds

If you need to move your child into a bed because you need the crib for the new baby, do it well before the due date. Try to present the idea as an exciting change (moving him into a "big boy" bed!) so that its about him rather than the baby—this will help your toddler feel pleased, not usurped. Depending on his age, you may opt for a crib that turns into a bed, or go straight to a single bed— safety rails that attach under the matress can be bought separately until he is used to the bed.

Minimize upheaval

If your child is ready, try to get any other major changes, such as toilet training, done before the arrival of new baby. This gives you less to do when the baby arrives, and avoids your child dealing with multiple upheavals all at once.

First impressions

When your child first meets his new sibling, it may be a good idea not to be cuddling her when he walks into the room. With free hands you can focus on him first, welcoming him with hugs and kisses. This will help him to feel secure and confident that you still love him and have time for him. Enjoy the first time your children meet—it is a magical moment, and one to cherish as a parent.

Little offerings

Ask your child if he'd like to give the baby a present or draw her a picture. He'll probably be eager to but, if not, don't force it. Maybe also buy a small present for him from the baby.

Your little helper

Make your child feel important and involved in family life by giving him a role as your helper. Ask him to tell you when the baby's crying or to get you a diaper when she needs changing. It'll nurture his caring side and he'll feel valued. Praise how he treats his sibling, for example: "she's happy because you're holding her so gently." Comments like this will boost his confidence and help to strengthen the bond between the children.

Time for two

Taking care of a newborn is time consuming, but it's important to have one-on-one time with your older child, perhaps when your baby is asleep, or when your partner can take her out for a walk. Your children should have time together, too. If your child is quite young you may need to keep a close eye since toddlers can be well-meaning but won't have any real concept of how gentle they must be.

> Spending quality, one-on-one time with your child should be a priority both before and after the baby is born.

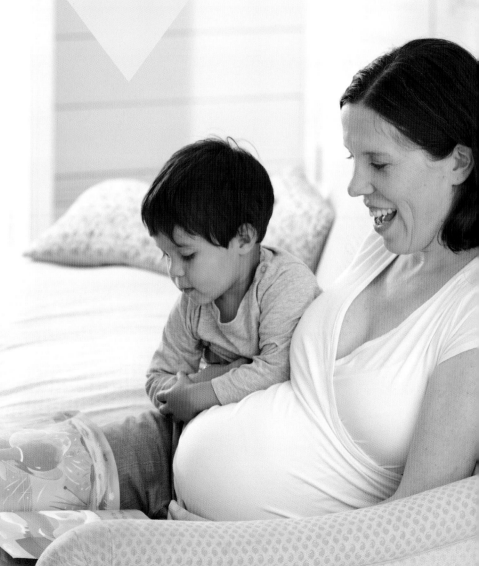

Hello, little baby—I'm going

1

2

3

…plus new baby makes four!

Your child will be curious about your growing belly and enjoy feeling the baby kick. Understanding her new role as a big sister helps her feel involved with (rather than displaced by) the new arrival, and feel that it is her baby, too.

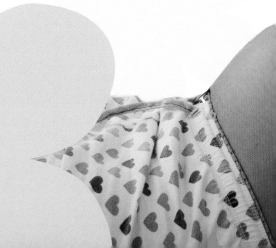

to be your big sister!

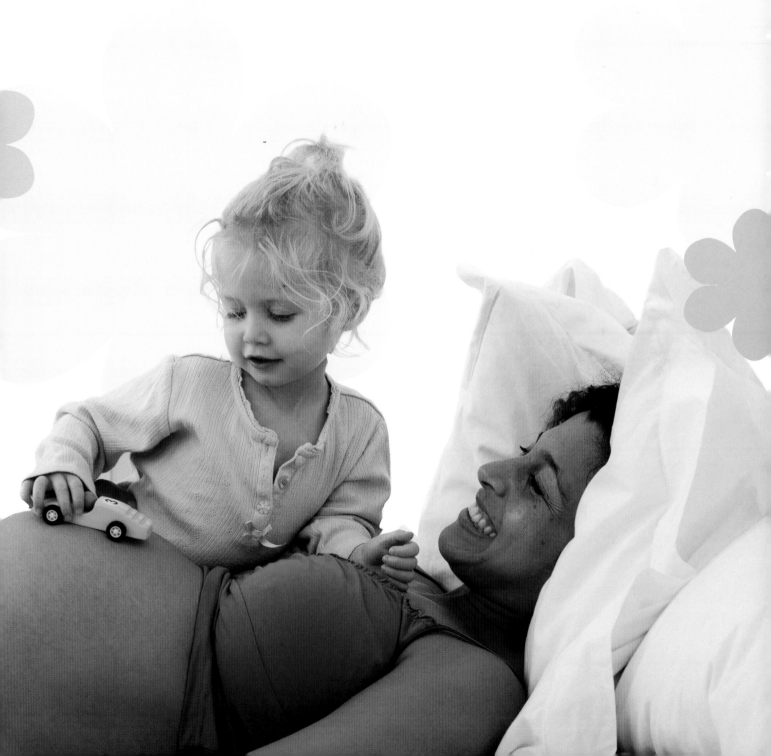

Who do I pick up *first?*

Taking care of a new baby is a challenge in itself, but what do you do if you've got an older child to take care of, too? Who needs to be your priority?

If you have a young child as well as a new baby, you really have your work cut out for you. There are **practical issues** to resolve such as how do you go to the bathroom and leave them both safely, and how to feed your baby when your older child wants you to play. If you need to pick up your older child from the babysitter or preschool, do you wake your sleeping baby or try to transfer her to a carriage still asleep? If both children cry at the same time, which should you go to first? There is also quite a bit of practical juggling to figure out, such as getting two children into a car or ready to go out for a walk, which can require a bit of planning. The key is not to try to do too much during this busy time.

Parents often worry about how an older child might feel when a new baby arrives: will she feel **left out or jealous**, and is it OK to leave her with baby? There are some tried-and-tested strategies to help you cope with the practicalities (see opposite). The first thing is don't try to do everything yourself. **Grandparents and relatives** can be very eager to help, a friend might have your older child on a playdate, or a neighbor could come over to watch your sleeping baby while you do the school run. Parents often end up taking care of one child more than the other, with Dad taking the older child while Mom has the baby. Swapping sometimes to give you **time with each child**, and a break from each set of needs, especially if you spend most of your time with your baby.

Helping your children get to know each other can be very enjoyable and can help **minimize jealousy**. Being fair is not easy and there will be phases in life when this is more and less important to them both, so don't worry if it isn't always possible.

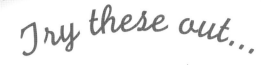

Try these out...

✳ If both children cry at once, go to the one whose
need is the greatest and can be most quickly resolved.
When everything is calm, cuddle both children.

✳ Wear your baby in a front pack or sling to free up your
hands while you do jobs, prepare a meal, or play with your toddler.

*When your toddler needs to burn off energy, go for a walk no matter
what the weather is. Put your baby in a front pack or carriage and ask
your toddler to help push. Take them to a park so she can run around.*

✳ Show your older child that her brother or sister
is a potential playmate rather than a rival. Say: "She loves to watch
what you're doing" and "She will want to join in one day."

✳ Install a safety
gate so you can keep your
toddler in a safe room when you
need to pop upstairs or go
to the bathroom.

For times when you must give your undivided attention to your
baby, such as breast-feeding, have a box of toddler supplies on hand
including toys, crayons, books, and games. Add a few inexpensive
new items to this every so often, to maintain her interest.

✳ *It's OK to ask your toddler to help you with simple baby care,
and it will make her feel involved. Always tell her how
much you value her help, and say thank you.*

✳ Get out your toddler's baby photographs to share with her. Tell her
stories about when she was a baby so she can remember that she was
fussed over also, and talk about how much more
she can do now that she is bigger.